THE MeNTaL EffecTs OF HEROIN

Anorexia Nervosa:
Starving for Attention

Child Abuse and Neglect:
Examining the Psychological Components

Conduct Unbecoming:
Hyperactivity, Attention Deficit, and Disruptive Behavior Disorders

Cutting the Pain Away:
Understanding Self-Mutilation

Drowning Our Sorrows:
Psychological Effects of Alcohol Abuse

Life Out of Focus:
Alzheimer's Disease and Related Disorders

The Mental Effects of Heroin

Psychological Disorders Related to Designer Drugs

Psychological Effects of Cocaine and Crack Addiction

Schizophrenia:
Losing Touch with Reality

Sibling Rivalry:
Relational Disorders Between Brothers and Sisters

Smoke Screen:
Psychological Disorders Related to Nicotine Use

Through a Glass Darkly:
The Psychological Effects of Marijuana and Hashish

The Tortured Mind:
The Many Faces of Manic Depression

When Families Fail:
Psychological Disorders Caused by Parent-Child Relational Problems

A World Upside Down and Backwards:
Reading and Learning Disorders

Senior Consulting Editor Carol C. Nadelson, M.D.
Consulting Editor Claire E. Reinburg

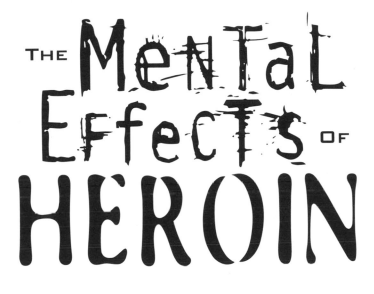

THE **MENTAL EFFECTS** OF **HEROIN**

Ann Holmes

CHELSEA HOUSE PUBLISHERS
Philadelphia

The ENCYCLOPEDIA OF PSYCHOLOGICAL DISORDERS *provides up-to-date information on the history of, causes and effects of, and treatment and therapies for problems affecting the human mind. The titles in this series are not intended to take the place of the professional advice of a psychiatrist or mental health care professional.*

Chelsea House Publishers
Editor in Chief: Stephen Reginald
Managing Editor: James D. Gallagher
Production Manager: Pamela Loos
Art Director: Sara Davis
Director of Photography: Judy L. Hasday
Senior Production Editor: Lisa Chippendale

Staff for THE MENTAL EFFECTS OF HEROIN
Editorial Assistants: Lily Sprague, Heather Forkos
Picture Researcher: Sandy Jones
Associate Art Director: Takeshi Takahashi
Designer: Brian Wible
Cover Design: Brian Wible

The ChelseaHouse World Wide Web site address is
http://www.chelseahouse.com

Library of Congress Cataloging-in-Publication Data

Holmes, Ann.
The Mental effects of heroin / by Ann Holmes.
  p. cm. — (The encyclopedia of psychological disorders)
Includes bibliographical references (p.   ) and index.
Summary:
ISBN 0-7910-4899-3 (hardcover)
 1. Heroin habit. I. Title. II. Series.
RC552.A5H38   1998
616.86'32—dc21   98-33640
                                                          CIP
                                                          AC

CONTENTS

PSYCHOLOGICAL DISORDERS AND THEIR EFFECT

CAROL C. NADELSON, M.D.
PRESIDENT AND CHIEF EXECUTIVE OFFICER,
The American Psychiatric Press

There are a wide range of problems that are considered psychological disorders, including mental and emotional disorders, problems related to alcohol and drug abuse, and some diseases that cause both emotional and physical symptoms. Psychological disorders often begin in early childhood, but during adolescence we see a sharp increase in the number of people affected by these disorders. It has been estimated that about 20 percent of the U.S. population will have some form of mental disorder sometime during their lifetime. Some psychological disorders appear following severe stress or trauma. Others appear to occur more often in some families and may have a genetic or inherited component. Still other disorders do not seem to be connected to any cause we can yet identify. There has been a great deal of attention paid to learning about the causes and treatments of these disorders, and exciting new research has taught us a great deal in the last few decades.

The fact that many new and successful treatments are available makes it especially important that we reject old prejudices and outmoded ideas that consider mental disorders to be untreatable. If psychological problems are identified early, it is possible to prevent serious consequences. We should not keep these problems hidden or feel shame that we or a member of our family has a mental disorder. Some people believe that something they said or did caused a mental disorder. Some people think that these disorders are "only in your head" so that you could "snap out of it" if you made the effort. This type of thinking implies that a treatment is a matter of willpower or motivation. It is a terrible burden for someone who is suffering to be blamed for their misery, and often people with psychological disorders are not treated compassionately. We hope that the information in this book will teach you about various mental illnesses.

The problems covered in the volumes in the ENCYCLOPEDIA OF PSYCHOLOGICAL DISORDERS were selected because they are of particular importance to young adults, because they affect them directly or because they affect family and friends. There are individual volumes on reading disorders, attention deficit and disruptive behavior disorders, and dementia—all of these are related to our abilities to learn and integrate information from the world around us. There are books on drug abuse that provide useful information about the effects of these drugs and treatments that are available for those individuals who have drug problems. Some of the books concentrate on one of the most common mental disorders, depression. Others deal with eating disorders, which are dangerous illnesses that affect a large number of young adults, especially women.

Most of the public attention paid to these disorders arises from a particular incident involving a celebrity that awakens us to our own vulnerability to psychological problems. These incidents of celebrities or public figures revealing their own psychological problems can also enable us to think about what we can do to prevent and treat these types of problems.

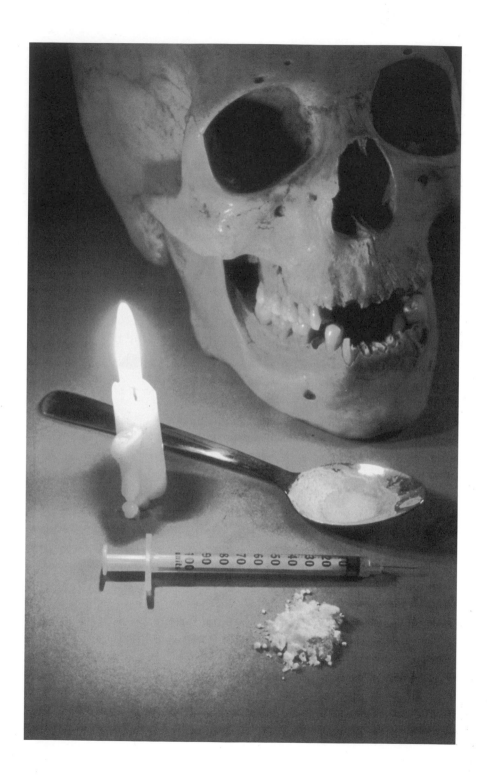

DRUG ABUSE AND HEROIN: AN OVERVIEW

One of the major public health problems facing the United States today is abuse of alcohol, tobacco, and other drugs. In 1962, about four million Americans admitted to having tried an illicit drug; by 1992 that number had climbed to almost 80 million.

The number of people addicted to or abusing various substances is enormous: more than 50 million people addicted to tobacco; over 18 million alcoholics or "problem drinkers"; more than five million people who admit to marijuana use more than once a week; over two million people addicted to cocaine; 750,000 or more people addicted to heroin; and up to half a million people who regularly use hallucinogens such as LSD (lysergic acid diethylamide), PCP (phencyclidine), and MDMA (methylenedioxymethamphetamine, also known as ecstasy). Staggering health care costs, crime, domestic violence, AIDS (acquired immunodeficiency syndrome), homelessness, and education and welfare problems are all related to our failure to deal adequately with substance abuse and dependence.

Although there are many drugs or substances that can cause serious physical, psychological, and social problems, in this book we will study heroin, a "hard" drug that is part of a group of drugs called opiates. Heroin use has never been higher in the United States, say those officials who closely monitor drug use in this country. "Heroin is a problem in Brattleboro, Vermont, and it is a problem in Yakima, Washington," Drug Enforcement Agency chief Thomas Constantine says. "There is no section of the country where heroin is not a threat." But increasing use of the drug is not limited to the United States, however. "Heroin has gone global, and there is no good news," International Narcotics Control Board official Bunsom Martin said in May 1997. The 1990s may well be the decade of opiate abuse.

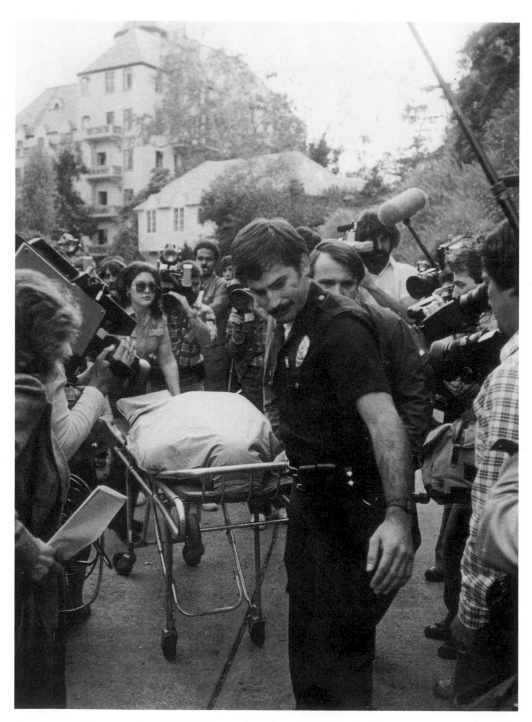

An emergency team removes the body of comedian John Belushi from the Chateau Marmont hotel in Los Angeles, where he died from an overdose of cocaine and heroin.

1

A DEADLY ADDICTION

John Belushi's death by accidental drug overdose stunned his fans. He had been a popular, successful young comedian with a bright future. Born in 1949 in a suburb of Chicago, Belushi had enjoyed popularity in high school. He was elected homecoming king and married his high school sweetheart, Judith Jacklin.

His father, an Albanian immigrant, owned two restaurants and had wanted to pass the family business down to John. John, however, was not interested. In February 1971 he joined Second City, a Chicago comedy troupe. He was its youngest performer, but he easily stole the show with acts like "Young Joe Cocker," which he later performed on *Saturday Night Live*. At this time he was also experimenting with a variety of drugs, including LSD, mushrooms, amphetamines, peyote, and acid. His popularity with Second City and National Lampoon led to his big career break as one of the original cast members of *Saturday Night Live*.

During the show's first year, John Belushi competed with Chevy Chase for fans and attention on the show. Both performers went through periods of increased cocaine abuse during the first season. When Chase married and left the show, Belushi no longer had to share the spotlight with him, but his drug intake increased during the second season. Over the next five years, Belushi starred in hit movies like *Animal House, 1941*, and *The Blues Brothers*. He also continued his self-destructive drug abuse, often going on binges of partying and drug-taking that could last for several days.

John spent the night of March 5, 1982, working on a movie script with friends. One of them gave him a "speedball," a powerful injection of cocaine and heroin. The mixture slowed down his heart rate and caused his heart to stop beating.

Although his sudden death shocked his fans, his friends, including fellow comedians Dan Ackroyd and Robin Williams, had been aware of his drug use. They simply hadn't comprehended the grave danger their friend was in; his pattern of drug use was similar to that of many Hollywood celebrities. John's death was a wake-up call for many.

■   ■   ■

Although her career was brief, many consider Janis Joplin to be one of the greatest blues/rock singers who ever lived. Her passionate, defiant spirit and her strong singing voice earned her national attention and popularity in the late 1960s, and she quickly rose to stardom. Heroin cut her career short just as it started to peak; she will forever be remembered as one of the drug's most talented victims.

Born in 1943 in Port Arthur, Texas, a small oil town, Janis tried hard to fit in with the other girls at Jefferson High School, but because she was overweight and had acne, her classmates teased her. Janis tried to act like she didn't care, but she was deeply hurt by their laughter. Her behavior became loud and flamboyant, and she would do anything to attract attention.

Her artistic career began to take off in her senior year of high school when she began both singing and selling her paintings. After graduating from Jefferson High School in 1960, she attended Lamar State College in Beaumont, Texas, for a year. She spent the summer of 1961 in California, first living in Los Angeles and then in Venice Beach, a popular area for "beatniks," the forerunners of the late-1960s hippie movement. The next year she attended the University of Texas at Austin. There she met more people who were also interested in experimental art and music. She began singing and playing the autoharp at lounges. But instead of drinking an occasional beer, Janis began downing six-packs. When she was drunk, her behavior became loud and antagonistic. She gave up painting, and she considered giving up music.

The following winter, Janis hitchhiked to San Francisco and spent the next two years traveling and performing. Doing drugs was a way for Janis to fit into the music scene in San Francisco. She became first a speed (amphetamines, or "uppers") addict and then, in 1964, a speed dealer. It was at this point that drugs began to take over her life.

Despite her addiction to speed, and later to heroin, Joplin's music career flourished. She became the lead singer of a group called Big Brother and the Holding Company. After gaining instant fame by taking the Monterey Pop Festival by storm in 1967, the group recorded its first

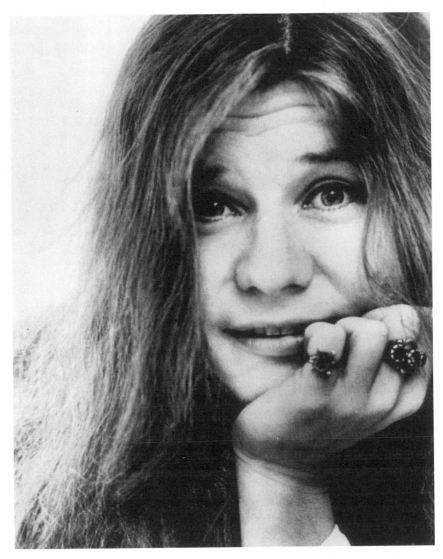

Singer Janis Joplin, whose strong blues-inspired singing style brought her to stardom before her death in 1970 of a heroin overdose.

album, *Cheap Thrills*, which sold well. However, Janis found it difficult to adjust to her newfound stardom. Though she was now famous, slim, and popular, Janis was still depressed. She continued to abuse drugs and alcohol. A few months after the release of *Cheap Thrills*, Janis left the band.

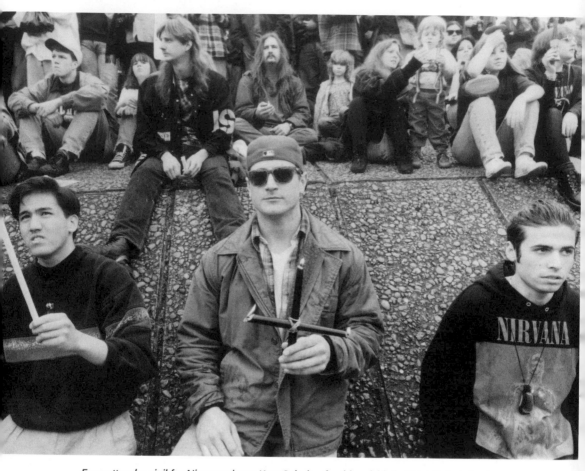

Fans attend a vigil for Nirvana singer Kurt Cobain after his suicide in 1994. Cobain had struggled with heroin abuse and related mental problems for years before his death.

In April 1970, after briefly performing with a group called the Kosmic Blues Band, Janis became the leader of the Full-Tilt Boogie Band. When they went on tour, she managed to give up heroin but still drank heavily before concerts. That summer she began to record her final album, *Pearl*. In August, she met Seth Morgan and fell in love. She felt happier and began to talk about marriage and family life.

But in September 1970, Janis began to do heroin again. A month later she collapsed in her hotel room and died of an accidental heroin overdose complicated by alcohol.

■   ■   ■

"I don't want my daughter to grow up and someday be hassled by kids at school . . . I don't want people telling her that her parents were junkies," Kurt Cobain told the reporter from the *Los Angeles Times* as he held his four-week-old baby girl in his lap in 1993. "I don't want to have anything to do with inciting drug use." Though he claimed to have put drugs behind him, many fans never stopped speculating about his rumored heroin addiction. Less than two years later, Cobain was dead of a self-inflicted gunshot to the head. His suicide is perhaps his most powerful statement about heroin's destructive capacities.

The lead singer of the alternative Seattle "grunge" band Nirvana, Kurt Cobain was born in the Washington logging town of Aberdeen in 1967. Always a frail child, Kurt suffered physically from bronchitis and recurring stomach pains, and emotionally from weathering the storms of his parents' rocky relationship. Their divorce when Kurt was eight shook him deeply, and he became sullen and withdrawn. As a teenager, Cobain enjoyed the music of bands like Aerosmith, Led Zeppelin, and Kiss; he first heard punk music in 1984. He dropped out of high school in 1985 and met Chris Novoselic a few months later. Together with drummer Dave Grohl, they formed a band and called it "Nirvana," taking the name from the Buddhist concept of eternal bliss. Their punk rock–influenced music was anything but blissful. Wearing ripped jeans and grungy plaid flannel shirts in concert, they would smash guitars and stage equipment in a destructive frenzy. Their music had a heavy-metal sound but still appealed to mainstream pop-rock fans.

Nevermind, their first album for a major record label, catapulted Nirvana into the spotlight almost overnight. Their hit "Smells Like Teen Spirit" was played continuously on MTV, and the band members were soon recognized everywhere they went. However, Kurt Cobain resented being a symbol of rebellion and disillusionment, "the crown prince of Generation X," to MTV fans and trendy teens—people with whom he felt he had nothing in common. He and his friends had once ridiculed popular rock stars; all of a sudden, he was one.

The unexpected fame and its accompanying pressures led to a period of increased drug use. Now that he was a big star, the heroin habit he developed was no longer just a dangerous personal choice—it sent a message to the youth of America, who looked to him as a trendsetter. He was aware of the profound influence his lyrics and actions could have on his millions of fans, and the idea scared him.

In 1992 he met and married Courtney Love, and together they had a daughter named Frances Bean Cobain. Having a family gave Kurt something to live for beyond his band and his music. After the birth of his daughter, Cobain claimed to be drug free, but rumors of his drug use persisted. He admitted to trying various drugs, blaming his stomach pains for his addiction to heroin. Nevertheless, he spoke out against teen drug addiction. He didn't want Nirvana to glamorize drug use the way some other bands do in their song lyrics and actions.

In March 1994 Kurt overdosed on painkillers and champagne in Rome and spent several hours in a coma. Doctors believed that the overdose was accidental, but less than a month later, his mind set on suicide, Cobain locked himself in his room with several weapons. This time, friends were able to talk him out of harming himself.

On April 8, 1994, Kurt Cobain's body was discovered on the floor of his apartment, by an electrician who had come to install an alarm system. He had shot himself in the head. His suicide note, written in red ink, lay nearby.

■   ■   ■

As the stories of John Belushi, Janis Joplin, and Kurt Cobain illustrate, heroin use can have devastating consequences. Heroin addiction does not just affect celebrities, however; the U.S. Office of National Drug Control Policy estimates that in the 1990s there are more than 800,000 "hard-core" heroin users—addicts—in the United States and that the number of "occasional" users increased from 210,000 in 1994 to 320,000 in 1995. And an annual survey by the National Household Survey on Drug Abuse, released in August 1998, reported that the number of teenagers using heroin for the first time had reached its highest level ever. Over 170,000 teens used heroin for the first time in 1996 (the last year data was available), up from 117,000 the year before. Plano, Texas, considered one of the nation's 10 safest cities, had 11 heroin-overdose deaths in 1997. In Orlando, Florida, 48 people died of heroin overdoses during 1995 and 1996; 10 of them were under age 21.

WHAT IS HEROIN?

Heroin is an illegal drug that is made from opium, the sap of the poppy plant *papaver somniferum*, or "sleep-inducing poppy." Today, the opium poppy is grown in small farms in remote regions of the world, with the majority of poppies grown either in a narrow 4,500-

Narcotics like heroin and morphine are made from the sap of the opium poppy, Papaver somniferum.

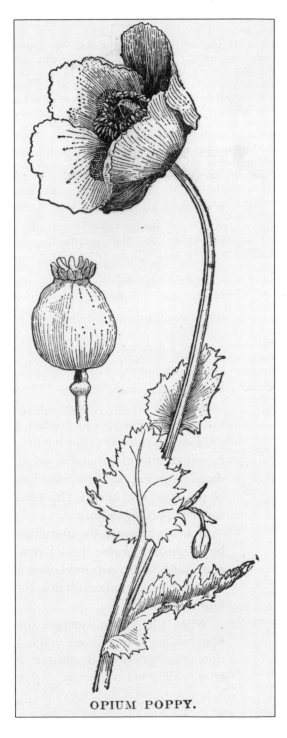

OPIUM POPPY.

mile stretch of mountains that extends across southern Asia from Turkey through Pakistan and Laos, or in Latin America (most notably Colombia). The plant flourishes in dry, warm climates.

About three months after poppy seeds are planted, brightly colored flowers bloom at the tips of greenish, tubular stems. As the petals fall away, they expose an egg-shaped seed pod. Inside the pod is an opaque, milky sap. This is opium in its crudest form.

The sap is harvested by slitting the pod vertically with parallel strokes using a special curved knife. As the sap oozes out, it turns darker and darker, forming a brownish-black gum. A farmer collects the gum with a scraping knife; allows it to harden into bricks, cakes, or balls; and wraps the opium sap in leaves or plastic. The farmer then sells the raw opium to a black-market merchant, who sends the resin to a morphine refinery. These illegal operations are often run near the farmer's home village. "Most traffickers do their morphine refining close to the poppy fields, since compact morphine bricks are much easier to smuggle than bundles of pungent, jelly-like opium," explains Alfred W. McCoy in *The Politics of Heroin.*

At the refinery, which may be little more than a sparsely equipped laboratory shrouded in a jungle thicket, the opium is mixed with lime in boiling water. Some organic material sinks to the bottom, but a white band forms on the surface: morphine. This morphine is drawn off; mixed with ammonia and reheated; filtered; and boiled down again until all that is left is a brown paste. This is called morphine base, and it is poured into molds and dried in the sun until it has the texture of dense modeling clay. Morphine base can be smoked in a pipe, or it can be processed into heroin. This entails a complicated series of steps in a well-equipped laboratory.

In making heroin, the morphine base is purified. However, this can be dangerous because the solvents that are used are highly explosive, and a careless chemist could cause an explosion that could level the laboratory. Purification results in a white, fluffy powder known as "number four" heroin.

When the heroin emerges from laboratories in places such as Bangkok and Hong Kong, it enters a complex chain of distribution. Big-time drug dealers usually deal in shipments of 20 to 100 kilograms, or kilos (a kilogram is a metric unit of measurement equal to 2.2 pounds). A New York drug lord, for example, might divide a bulk shipment into wholesale lots of one to ten kilos for sale to pushers that make up his distribution network. Dealing drugs is a big, expensive business. A kilo of Southeast Asian heroin cost $100,000 to $120,000 in 1997, according to the Drug Enforcement Administration (DEA). By dividing the kilo of heroin into small bags valued at between $5 and $100, which are peddled on city streets, the value of a kilogram of heroin is increased more than 10 times.

Not many years ago virtually all the heroin sold on America's streets was so heavily diluted that it was only about 10 percent pure. The purity of heroin has risen sharply in the 1990s as dealers try to expand their market beyond those addicts who inject heroin into their veins with hypodermic needles. Today, heroin purchased on the street may be 50 to 60 percent pure. Higher purity means "you can inhale it, you can smoke it, you can get high without the threat of AIDS or those nasty intravenous needles," DEA administrator Thomas Constantine told the *Washington Post* in 1997.

It takes approximately 10 tons of opium to make one ton of heroin. In 1996, the worldwide opium output was 430 tons, which was processed into approximately 38 tons of heroin. About half of that was intended to be smuggled into North America, with 12 tons going to the United States.

Heroin use is on the rise in the United States, according to Barry McCaffrey, the director of the Office of National Drug Control Policy. His office's winter 1997 report, *Pulse Check: National Trends in Drug Abuse*, noted:

> The rise in the availability of higher purity heroin and increased use that began in Northeastern cities in the early 1990s has now reached all areas of the country. . . . [S]ome sources report increases in the number of heroin users entering treatment facilities as well as increased numbers of emergency room episodes and overdose deaths related to heroin. Law enforcement sources report that heroin is part of both the street drug trade and the club drug market and is being sold by a wider range of dealers who are likely to sell both heroin and cocaine. In short, heroin has made a comeback almost everywhere, and it is no longer confined to older addicts from another generation of drug users. Many sources report that it is once again a flourishing part of the drug culture in their areas.

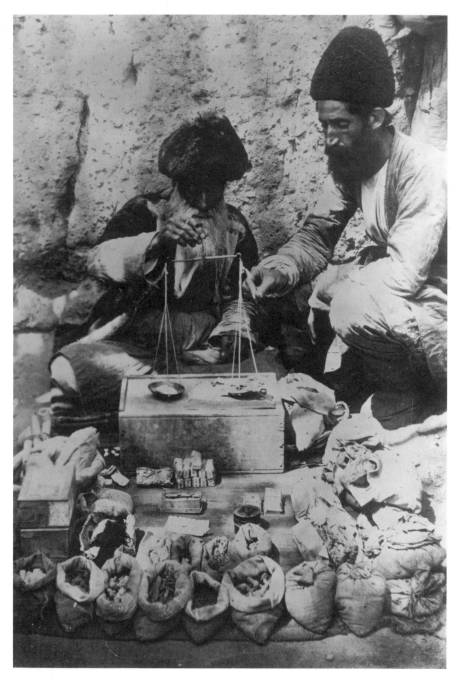

Opium sellers weigh the drug in an open-air marketplace in Persia (present-day Iran). Opium poppies were first cultivated in the Middle East over 5,000 years ago.

A HISTORY OF OPIUM USE

Throughout history, the opium poppy, *papaver somniferum*, has played a major role in a number of different cultures. The painkilling and calming properties of the poppy's extract, opium, were first recognized more than 5,000 years ago. The ancient Sumerians began cultivating the poppy in lower Mesopotamia (in present-day Iraq) around 3400 B.C. They called it *hul gil*, meaning "the joy plant." Later, the Assyrians and the Babylonians learned how to collect the juice of the poppy, and used it in potions and medical remedies. They passed this knowledge on to the ancient Egyptians, who grew the poppies in large fields near their capital city, Thebes, and called their opium preparations *opium thebacium*. The opium trade flourished around 1300 B.C. during the reign of the pharaohs Thutmose IV, Akhenaton, and Tutankhamen (later known as King Tut). The trade route included Phoenicia (present-day Lebanon), the island of Crete, mainland Greece, Carthage (a city in North Africa), and the coastal cities of Europe. The poppy became so important in Egypt as a remedy that the ancient pharaohs were entombed with both the plants and the equipment to recover opium from the poppy bulb.

In Greek mythology, the poppy and opium were regarded as gifts from the gods. On the island of Cyprus, surgical-quality culling knives were crafted to harvest opium. The people of Cyprus cultivated, smoked, and traded opium before the legendary city of Troy was sacked by the Greeks around 1750 B.C. Use of the poppy continued to spread, thanks to the conquests of Alexander the Great. Around 330 B.C. his Greek armies spread opium use into Persia (present-day Iran) and India.

Hippocrates (460–377 B.C.), the Greek physician who is called "the father of medicine," wrote about the usefulness of opium—both as a narcotic and in treating diseases. He prescribed it frequently as a remedy. About 600 years

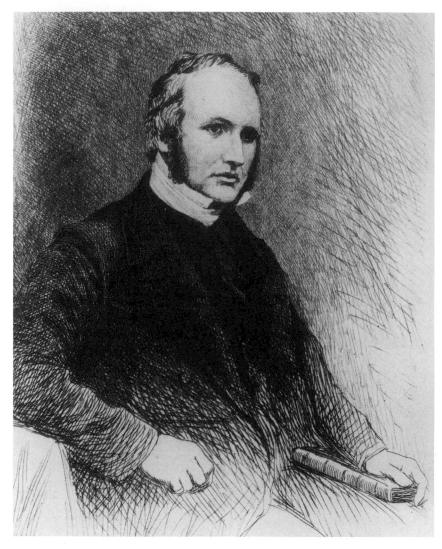

Alexander Wood developed the hypodermic syringe, and discovered that when morphine was administered with a needle, its effects were felt more quickly and were more potent.

later, a Greek physician named Galen created a standard recipe for preparation of opium. He called it *mithridate*.

By A.D. 400, opium from the Egyptian poppy fields at Thebes was introduced to China by Arab traders. By the seventh century, the Turkish and Islamic cultures of western Asia learned that opium's effects could be heightened if the poppy's juices were dried and smoked. This practice soon spread to China and India, as did the practice of creating mild opium-based drinks to be used as painkillers for minor ailments—not unlike the way aspirin is used today.

By the 11th century, doctors in the Middle East had recorded that as a person took opium over time, larger amounts were needed to produce the same effect. This indicated that the person's body had become tolerant to the drug. These Arab scientists also wrote that continued use of the drug "degenerates," "corrupts," and "weakens the mind."

In Europe during this time, use of opium nearly disappeared because of the powerful Catholic Church, which had strict prohibitions on medicine during the medieval period. But early in the 16th century, a Swiss physician named Paracelsus developed an opium-based medication he called *laudanum*, which he claimed could cure any pain-producing disease and even rejuvenate people who were close to death. His preparation, which also included citrus juice and powdered gold, quickly became the most popular medication of its day and was widely used—and abused.

By 1606, ships chartered by Queen Elizabeth I were instructed to purchase the finest Indian opium and transport it back to England. In 1680, an English apothecary (a name for an early pharmacist), Thomas Sydenham, introduced Sydenham's laudanum, a compound of opium, sherry wine, and herbs. His pills, and other opium-based medications of the time, became popular remedies for numerous ailments.

In 1803, Friedrich Sertuerner, a scientist from Paderborn, Germany, discovered the active ingredient of opium by dissolving it in acid and then neutralizing it with ammonia. What he found was a crystal alkaloid, an organic compound that contains nitrogen. He named this element *morphine*, after the ancient Greeks' mythological god of sleep and dreams, Morpheus. As a result of Sertuerner's discovery, physicians believed that opium had finally been perfected and "tamed," and morphine was lauded as "God's own medicine" for its reliability, long-lasting painkilling effects, and safety. In 1827 E. Merck & Company of Darmstadt, Germany, began commercial manufacture of morphine. The development of the hypodermic syringe in the 1840s changed the way that morphine was used. In 1843 Dr. Alexander Wood of Edinburgh discovered that when morphine was injected with a needle, its effect on his patients was instantaneous and three times as powerful. By 1845, Great Britain was importing over 20,000 pounds of opium a year.

The 19th century saw an increased use of opium-based medications, morphine, and opium for recreational use—literary figures such as John Keats, Samuel Taylor Coleridge, and Edgar Allan Poe used the drug occasionally just for the "high." But this trend was not without its critics. In 1822 Thomas DeQuincy published an autobiographical account of opium addiction, *Confessions of an English Opium Eater*. His book, which described how he went from the use of laudanum for medicinal purposes to an addictive craving for the drug, captivated the public and physicians. He documented how the body develops tolerance to the drug and the symptoms of withdrawal when the user attempts to stop taking the drug. However, people continued to use laudanum for a variety of ailments.

OPIUM LEADS TO WAR

The Dutch had introduced the practice of smoking opium to the Chinese in the 18th century, when they began exporting shipments of Indian opium to China and Southeast Asia. By 1750, the British East India Company had assumed control of the Indian opium trade, and the British began to market opium aggressively in the large market that China offered. The British East India Company had established a monopoly on the opium trade by 1793, and poppy growers in India were forbidden to sell opium to competing trading companies.

The opium trade with China was an extremely lucrative business for the British, bringing millions of dollars into the country's economy each year. By 1820 more than 300 tons of pure opium were imported into China, and in 10 years annual imports approached 2,000 tons. Millions of Chinese were becoming addicted to opium.

The Chinese government, attempting to break the drug's hold on the country, banned opium in 1838. Foreign traders were ordered to surrender their opium, and the new Chinese policy called for users to be executed. With the opium trade endangered, the British sent warships to the coast of China, and the Opium War of 1839 began. When the Chinese lost the war with Britain after three years of fighting, they were forced to sign the Treaty of Nanking, which required them to pay a large fine to the British, cede control of the port of Hong Kong to Great Britain, and submit to England's commercial interests. As a result, opium imports to China doubled by 1852.

In 1856, in an effort to gain additional trade privileges, the British and French renewed hostilities against China in the Second Opium War.

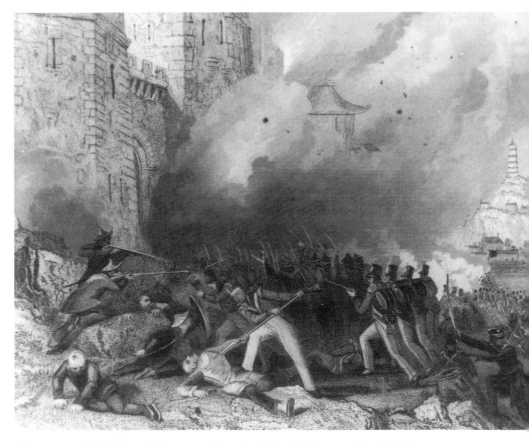

The capture of Chin-Q'iang-Fu in 1842, during the Opium War between Great Britain and China. The English victory in the three-year war forced the Chinese to end a ban on opium trade and use, and opened new ports to the West.

Defeated again, China was forced to pay another indemnity and open 11 additional ports to Western trade.

A NEW DRUG APPEARS: HEROIN

In 1874, an English researcher, C. R. Wright, boiled morphine over a stove. He called the resulting substance diacetylmorphine. However, this new substance remained unknown to most physicians and the general public for the next 25 years. In 1898, Heinrich Dreser, a chemist and researcher who worked for the Bayer Company of Elberfeld, Germany, discovered that diluting morphine with acetic acid and then boiling the compound down produces a drug that is more potent than morphine. Dreser, who had also worked on developing aspirin for Bayer, believed that his new drug compound did not include the side effects of morphine: nausea, psychological impairment, and dependence. Bayer began production of diacetylmorphine and came up with a new trade name: heroin.

Soon, however, the company's researchers realized that heroin produced the same dependence and symptoms of morphine and affected its users faster than any other opiate. Bayer immediately stopped promoting the product. However, the company continued to distribute it for several years. This was long enough for others to learn how to duplicate Bayer's recipe for the potent new narcotic.

NARCOTIC USE IN THE UNITED STATES

In the United States, laudanum was widely available and used for common ailments, and morphine had become a popular painkiller by the mid-19th century. In fact, overuse of morphine on the battlefields of the Civil War led to addictions, called the "army disease," in many wounded soldiers. And beginning in the 1850s, thousands of Chinese immigrants entered the United States to help build the railroads and work the mines in the West. These immigrants brought with them the practice of smoking opium, and soon the "opium dens" of West Coast cities such as San Francisco became notorious. As a result, imports of opium into the United States increased twentyfold between 1830 and 1870.

After the Civil War ended in 1865, government authorities on the West Coast began to worry about the effects of narcotic addiction and began to enact anti-opium laws. Also underlying this legislation was strong anti-Chinese sentiment among the white settlers of the West. In 1874 San Francisco banned opium smoking within the city limits, confining it to the Chinatown neighborhood. In 1883 and in 1890 the Congress of the United States imposed tariffs on opium and morphine. By the turn of the century, the U.S. government had recognized the danger of narcotics. In 1905, Congress banned opium use in the United States, and two years later the Pure Food and Drug Act was passed, requiring that the contents of patent medicines—which often included opiates or alcohol as their active ingredient—must be labeled by pharmaceutical companies. As a result, the availability of opiates declined significantly. In 1909, the importation of opium was completely banned in the United States, in preparation for an international conference on drug use later that year.

When the International Opium Commission convened in Shanghai in 1909, the U.S. delegates, Dr. Hamilton Wright and Episcopal Bishop Henry Brent, argued that narcotic distribution should be restricted worldwide. The conference participants, which included England and many other European nations, agreed. At the Hague Conference three years later, specific recommendations were made to further the goals of the Shanghai Conference.

America's response to these conferences was to pass the Harrison Narcotics Act, aimed at curbing cocaine and narcotic distribution and use. However, the law did not ban heroin because at the time Congress did not realize its addictive properties. This law, and increased enforcement practices, brought a rapid decrease in American consumption of opiates and in the number of users, especially those who only occasionally used the drug.

For people with serious addictions to opium, morphine, or cocaine, however, there were no treatment programs available. Trying to "kick the habit" was nearly impossible alone, and drug users turned to a still-legal alternative: heroin. In 1924, the U.S. Treasury Department's Narcotics Division (the first federal drug agency) banned heroin distribution. This forced addicts to buy on the black market from street dealers and led to a criminal underworld specializing in the distribution of narcotics.

HEROIN AVAILABILITY TODAY

International smuggling of opium was disrupted during World War II. Because of the Japanese conquest of China, Burma, and parts of Southeast Asia, opium trade routes were blocked and the flow of opium from India and Persia to the West was cut off. The French, afraid of losing their monopoly on opium production, encouraged Hmong farmers in the Southeast Asian highlands to expand their opium production.

In the years after World War II—the early years of the Cold War—the United States adopted a foreign policy designed to contain the spread of Communism around the world. In Southeast Asia, one of the most volatile areas, this involved forging alliances with tribes and warlords inhabiting the areas of the "Golden Triangle," a region including Laos, Thailand, and Myanmar (formerly Burma). In order to maintain their

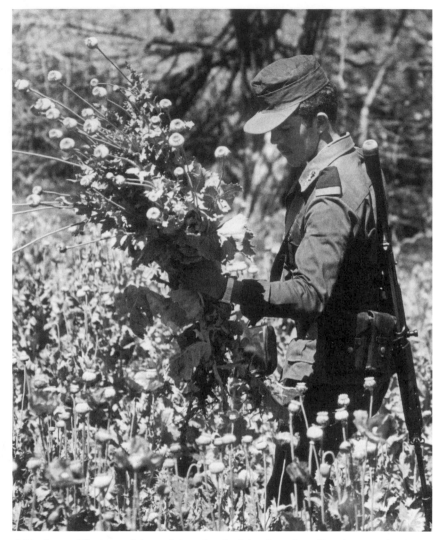

A Mexican soldier, part of the anti-drug Condor brigade, collects illegal poppy plants during a sweep of the state of Sinaloa in an attempt to curb the growth of Mexico's share of the world heroin market.

relationships with these nations, the United States and France supplied ammunition, arms, and air transport. All were used for the production and sale of opium. The result: an explosion in the illegal flow of heroin into the United States. In addition, U.S. involvement in the Vietnam conflict exposed many young Americans to a cheap and easily available supply of the drug. These factors resulted in a rash of new addictions. In the late 1950s there were approximately 100,000 heroin addicts in the United States; by 1975 that number had reached 750,000 and was still growing.

By 1978 the United States was making an all-out effort to stop heroin smugglers. An attempt in conjunction with the Mexican government to eliminate one source of raw opium—by spraying poppy fields with Agent Orange—was termed a success as the amount of the heroin nick-named "Mexican mud" in the U.S. drug market declined. However, in response another source of heroin was found in an area called the "Golden Crescent" (Iran, Afghanistan, and Pakistan).

In 1993, the Thai army, with support from the U.S. Drug Enforcement Agency, launched an operation to destroy thousands of acres of opium poppies in fields of the Golden Triangle region. That same year, popular young actor River Phoenix died outside a Hollywood nightclub from an overdose of heroin and cocaine. A year later, Kurt Cobain died of a heroin-related suicide. Their deaths brought the growing problem of heroin abuse to the forefront.

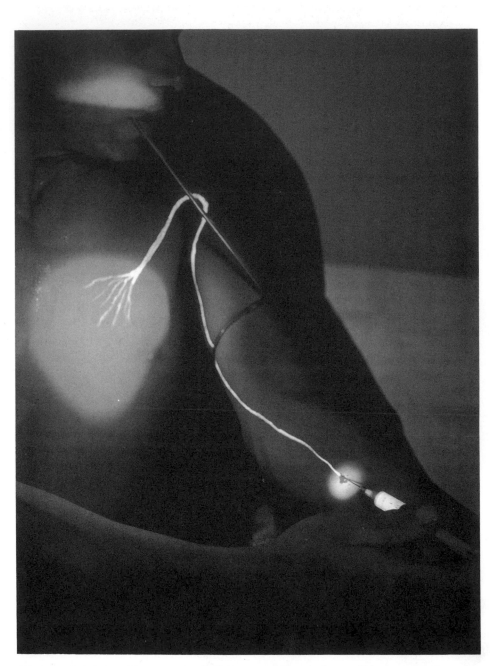

When heroin is injected into a user's vein, it is transported to the heart within moments, then pumped in the blood to all parts of the body.

3

THE PHYSICAL EFFECTS
OF OPIOIDS

Because "substance" refers to any kind of specific physical material, a substance-related disorder is a problem caused by introducing something into the body. This might be a legal product such as alcohol, caffeine, or cigarettes, an illegal drug like heroin or cocaine, a medication (such as a prescription pain killer), or a poison (such as lead).

People take substances to change the way they feel: to reduce pain, to stimulate the body, to induce relaxation, or to produce feelings of intoxication. Intoxication is the effect that a user experiences when taking a drug like heroin. The most common effects of intoxication include:

- Difficulties in perception (basically knowing what is or isn't real)
- Difficulty sleeping/wakefulness
- Impairment to attention span and judgment
- Disruptive behavior, and
- Awkward physical movement.

The effects of intoxication—the way a drug makes a person feel—differ from substance to substance and person to person. The frequency of drug use, the amount of the drug that is taken, and even user expectations of how the drug will make them feel can influence the drug's intoxicating effects.

When a person cannot stop using a substance such as alcohol, cocaine, or heroin, we say they are addicted, or substance dependent. A person who is addicted to heroin, for example, will continue to abuse the drug despite the significant problems that taking heroin causes. Addiction to heroin combines two problems: physical dependence and psychological dependence. Physical dependence means that the person's body has become so used to the drug that unpleasant physical symptoms will occur if it is withdrawn suddenly.

Psychological dependence means that the drug user has a powerful craving to use the drug, even if there is no physical drive to do so.

Tolerance is a need for greater and greater amounts of the drug to achieve the intoxication, or "high." A heroin user who has a high tolerance for the drug needs to take larger amounts to achieve the same "buzz" feeling experienced on first use. In time, many drug abusers develop such a high tolerance for their drug that they can take an amount that would kill a nonuser. Many drug-related deaths occur when first-time users take a dose that is too high.

Withdrawal occurs when a person's body has become so used to a drug that it adapts chemically, becoming dependent on the drug. When that person stops taking the drug and amounts of the substance in the body decline, unpleasant symptoms occur. These can be both mental and physical and may include severe muscle cramps, nausea, convulsions, and hallucinations. The symptoms of withdrawal can be so unpleasant that the user will continue to take the drug just to avoid them.

THE EFFECTS OF HEROIN

Heroin is an illegal substance that is part of a group of drugs called opiates. Other drugs in this family, derived from the opium poppy, include morphine and codeine, both of which are effective painkillers and have many medical uses. There are also a number of synthetic opiates that are used as painkillers. These include pethidine and methadone, which is often prescribed for heroin and opiate addiction. Collectively opiates and synthetic opiates are called opioids.

Opioids cause people to feel drowsy, warm, and content. They also relieve stress and discomfort by creating a relaxed detachment from pain, desires, and activity. As well as killing pain, moderate doses of pure opioids produce a range of mild effects. They depress, or slow, the activity of the body's central nervous system, affecting such reflexes as coughing, breathing, and heart rate. They also cause widening of the blood vessels, which gives the feeling of warmth.

The effects of heroin are more immediately powerful than the effects of any other opiate. Within seconds of injection into a vein, the user experiences a pleasant surge of feelings through his or her body. Although the user feels peaceful, this can be very dangerous: if the dose is too high, this rush of feeling can be so intense that the body slips into a coma or forgets to breathe, leading to death. The chance of an over-

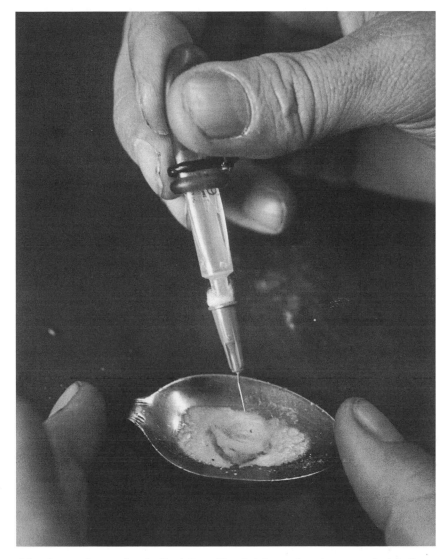

A heroin user draws a "cooked" solution of heroin into a syringe to prepare for injection. Sharing contaminated needles or syringes can spread blood-borne diseases such as HIV (AIDS) and hepatitis among addicts.

dose is greatly increased if other depressant drugs such as alcohol or tranquilizers are being used at the same time.

In a few minutes, the intense feelings fade. This is followed by a few hours of gradually decreasing sensation that are usually accompanied

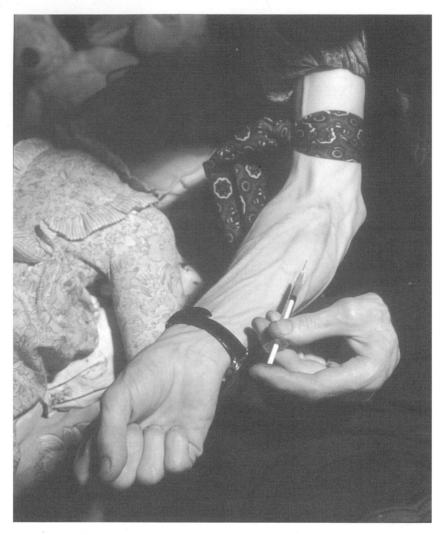

Frequent injection of heroin can cause a user's veins to become damaged or collapse. The drug also reduces appetite, leading to malnutrition and unhealthy weight loss.

by feelings of sleepiness, or lethargy. Regular users say that heroin makes them feel "peaceful" or "protected"—however, these feelings are illusory and do not last once the drug's effects wear off.

Because heroin acts on the nervous system, a user's pulse and breathing rates are slowed and his or her blood pressure drops. The physical symptoms of someone who is high on heroin include poor coordination, slurred speech, and slowed reactions. Users' pupils are constricted and eyes are watery, and their faces may be flushed. Often, heroin causes itching that may lead the user to scratch distractedly while feeling the drug's intoxicating effects. Nausea is another common side effect of heroin use, especially in first-time users.

HOW HEROIN IS TAKEN

Heroin, and other opioids in powder form, are commonly dissolved in water, heated, and injected into a vein to maximize the effect. At one time, intravenous injection was the most common way for users to take the drug; however, injection can be deadly. Intravenous drug users have a high risk for the human immunodeficiency virus (HIV), the virus that causes AIDS, as well as other diseases such as hepatitis, because users often share needles that have been tainted with contaminated blood.

Today, it is common for a user to sniff, or snort, heroin powder, or to smoke the powder (this method is sometimes called "chasing the dragon"). Although the effects of heroin occur nearly as quickly when the drug is snorted or smoked, it produces a less-intense effect than when it is injected.

The drug has many common street nicknames, including "lady," "white girl," "horse," "black tar," "brown sugar," "smack," "H," "harry," "skag," and "junk."

THE DANGERS OF HEROIN USE

Heroin use is dangerous because it can permanently change the way a person's body works. This is not the only damage the drug can cause physically, however. As explained earlier in this chapter, long-term use of opioids causes the user to develop a tolerance to the drug's effects. In order to achieve the same degree of euphoria, larger and larger doses must be taken. This often leads to a fatal overdose. In addition, drug abusers who have abstained from using the drug for some time, perhaps trying to quit, may not realize that their tolerance for heroin has decreased. If one of these users take the drug again, it would be easy to overdose by taking the same amount of the drug used before quitting.

When the drug is being used regularly, a negative reaction will occur about 12 hours after the effects of the last dose wear off. These withdrawal symptoms include muscle aches, sweating and chills, convulsions and muscular spasms, and delirium or hallucinations. Usually the symptoms peak within two days, and ease in three to five days, but feelings of weakness, insomnia, or a loss of well-being may persist for weeks or months.

There are two ways to withdraw from the drug. The first, cutting off all drug use abruptly, is often called "quitting cold turkey." This produces the strongest withdrawal symptoms. Another is to be weaned from the drug gradually by using decreasing doses. This lessens the suffering from withdrawal symptoms but spreads them over a longer period of time.

The symptoms of withdrawal are affected by the amount of time a user has been taking the drug, the amount of the drug that he or she has taken, and other factors. A person who for many years was a heavy user of heroin will have a harder time withdrawing from the drug than a person who has used it a few times over a one-month period.

In addition, prolonged usage can cause physical damage to the body that is not directly a result of the drug itself. As mentioned earlier, heroin addicts often share needles. If one of the users has a disease that can be spread through infected blood, such as HIV or hepatitis, passing that user's dirty needle also passes the disease. Other diseases that can be passed through dirty needles include tetanus, septicemia (blood poisoning that can result in the loss of a limb or even death), and endocarditis (an infection of the heart valve). Another problem common among heroin addicts is collapsed or damaged veins from the regular injections of the drug. In addition, the injection itself can kill the user: if the addict accidentally injects some air into a vein, he or she may die in a few seconds when the air bubble reaches the brain.

Heroin use reduces a person's appetite. This often leads to malnutrition and its resulting physical problems. Prolonged use of opiates also has been shown to reduce the body's effectiveness for fighting illness.

Among the dangers of using heroin or other illicit drugs is that users can never be sure what they are putting into their bodies. Because heroin sold at street level has often been cut, or diluted, with other substances such as sugar, caffeine, flour, or talcum powder, there is always a risk of using impure drugs. Sometimes, quinine or other drugs are used as cutting agents, and this can increase the possibility of accidental overdose.

The increasing cost of satisfying a heroin dependence can lead to money problems. Addicts often turn to criminal activity to get the money to support a drug habit.

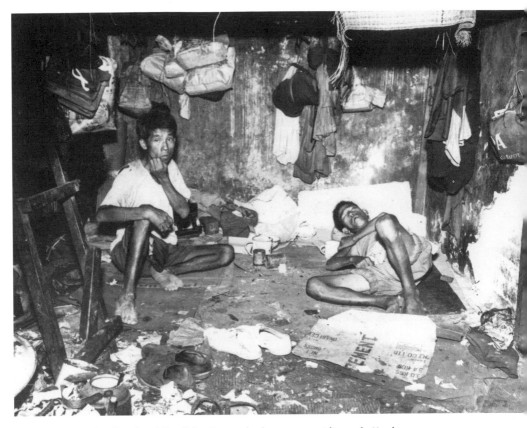

Emaciated and dirty heroin addicts living in squalor in a tenement house in Kowloon, Hong Kong.

HEROIN'S PROBLEMS ARE WORLDWIDE

Although a large percentage of the world's heroin is shipped to the United States, abuse of heroin and other drugs is a worldwide problem. For example, more than 150,000 residents of St. Petersburg, Russia, are believed to be hooked on heroin, cocaine, LSD, or other illicit substances.

"There are several reasons why drug use is increasing," Detective Alexander Smirnov, a member of that city's drug enforcement administration, explained in an Associated Press news report from 1996. "First, many people live in very bad conditions. Second, they don't understand the dangers of using drugs. And third, the government is not showing much concern about the problem."

THE DANGER OF SMUGGLING HEROIN

Heroin is a dangerous drug, and using it can lead to illness, disease, and death. Heroin can also be dangerous to those people who are caught attempting to smuggle the drug from one country to another, or to sell the drug in the United States, as a former award-winning television journalist discovered a few years ago.

Steven Roye, an Emmy Award–winning reporter for WWOR-TV in New Jersey, was arrested in 1994 at Don Muang International Airport, Bangkok, Thailand, as he was preparing to board a plane for Amsterdam. When his belongings were searched, police discovered six and a half pounds of heroin sewn into the lining of one of his suitcases.

When he was arraigned, Roye pleaded innocent, telling the court that he had been forced to carry the heroin while researching drug trafficking links between Thailand and the United States for an investigative report. He told the judge that Thai criminals had threatened to harm his family if he didn't carry the heroin for them. Several months later, on the advice of his lawyers, Roye changed his plea to guilty.

Under the law in Thailand, drug traffickers automatically receive the death penalty. However, no foreigner has been executed in decades for smuggling drugs, and Roye's lawyers believed he could expect a 25-year sentence. But at the trial in October 1995, the Thai court reduced Roye's sentence from execution to life in prison because he had changed his plea to guilty.

"I'm totally outraged," Roye said as he was led from the court. "I'm in total disbelief. A life sentence for what? Even if I had done it, I didn't deserve life. You should give a life sentence to killers.

"I was totally gone when they read the sentence," he continued. "I expected I might get 25, 30, or even 35 years, but I never expected a life sentence."

With no parole possible, Steven Roye's best hope is an eventual pardon from Thailand's constitutional monarch, King Bhumipol Adulyadej, who has occasionally pardoned foreigners jailed for drug offenses after they have served just a few years of their sentence.

Drugs are not difficult to find in St. Petersburg if you have the right contacts, according to one addict, Volodya. He is a regular customer at a produce market that is known locally as a place to buy drugs and the ingredients to make them. "I buy the raw poppy plant at the market, always from the same guy. He just sells it right in there where they sell fruits, potatoes and vegetables. He sells it to me in glassfulls," Volodya told the Associated Press reporter. "I use one glass a day. Glasses usually cost about 20,000 rubles each, but I get a discount, since I'm such a good customer."

It takes Volodya about 40 minutes in his kitchen to convert the poppy essence to heroin. Russian heroin (known as "black") is much different from what U.S. users would call heroin. "Pure heroin is far too expensive for Russian users," Detective Smirnov explained. "Russian heroin is a mixture of brown and white heroin, and is made by the user himself from poppy plants and other ingredients. . . . The more additives, the less expensive the doses end up being, so people add all kinds of impurities until the end product is a dangerous, dirty blend."

Volodya is unemployed. In order to support his habit, he periodically disappears for a few days to "earn money." Where he goes and what he does are a well-kept secret. He leaves his four-year-old daughter with his parents. His daughter's mother, also an addict, disappeared 18 months before.

"Sometimes I wish I could quit," Volodya says. "But the treatment I know of is expensive, and has to be paid at once. I don't know if I'll ever be able to stop."

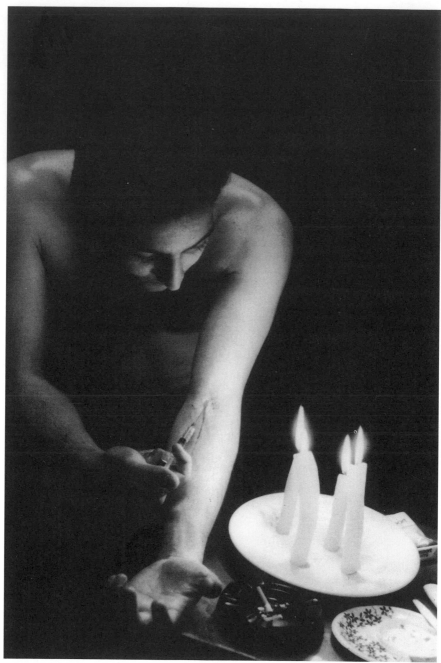

 Heroin's effects are not only physical; the drug also causes both short- and long-term mental problems for the user.

4

PSYCHOLOGICAL DISORDERS CAUSED BY HEROIN ABUSE

I n addition to the many physical problems caused by abuse of heroin and other opioids, the drugs have both short- and long-term mental effects. These psychological effects have been categorized as "substance-related disorders" in the American Psychiatric Association's *Diagnostic and Statistical Manual of Mental Disorders*, fourth edition (*DSM-IV*), the major reference work in the field of psychology.

Substance-related disorders are psychological disorders that occur as a result of a person taking a drug (including alcohol and tobacco) or medication or ingesting a toxin. The *DSM-IV* separates drugs into 11 categories. Opioids is one; the others are alcohol, amphetamines, caffeine, cannabis (marijuana), cocaine, hallucinogens, inhalants, nicotine, PCP, and sedatives. Sometimes, prescribed or over-the-counter medicines can also cause substance-related disorders, the *DSM-IV* notes. And exposure to toxins, such as lead-based paint, carbon monoxide, or gasoline fumes, may also lead to psychological disorders. In most cases, the symptoms of a substance-related disorder disappear when the person is no longer exposed to the drug, medication, or toxin causing the disorder. However, in some cases the disorder will persist for several weeks, and some form of treatment may be necessary.

The *DSM-IV* divides substance-related disorders into two groups: substance-use disorders and substance-induced disorders. There are two substance-use disorders, substance dependence and substance abuse. The substance-induced disorders include intoxication and withdrawal, which were discussed earlier in this book, as well as intoxication-delirium disorder, opioid-induced psychotic disorder, mood disorders, sexual dysfunction, and sleep disorders.

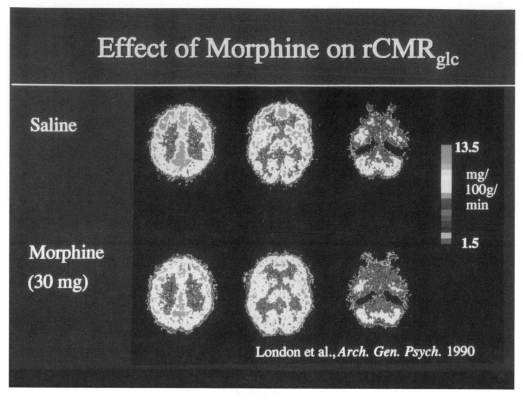

These scans show the depressant effects of morphine on the brain. The subject injected with the morphine solution shows lower levels of brain activity.

OPIOID DEPENDENCE AND ABUSE

✵ With opioid dependence, the user is addicted and continues to take the drug despite any problems that its use causes. Most users with opioid dependence have high tolerance and will experience withdrawal symptoms if use of heroin is stopped abruptly. A psychologist diagnosing opioid dependence must note symptoms that reflect uncontrollable and prolonged use of heroin or another opioid, other than for a legitimate medical purpose. If the patient being studied does have a medical condition that requires treatment with an opioid-based medicine, such as cough suppressants or an anti-diarrhea medication, opioid dependence may be diagnosed if the substance is used in doses greatly exceeding the amount needed for pain relief.

Persons with opioid dependence tend to develop such regular patterns of compulsive drug use that daily activities are typically planned around obtaining and administering the drug. Opioids are usually purchased on the illegal market. However, they may also be obtained from physicians by faking or exaggerating general medical problems or by receiving simultaneous prescriptions from several different doctors.

Opioid dependence is commonly associated with a history of drug-related crimes, such as possession or distribution of drugs, burglary, or robbery. People with opioid dependence are especially at risk to develop brief depressive symptoms and episodes of mild to moderate depression. Depression is characterized by an inability to concentrate, insomnia, and feelings of extreme sadness, dejection, and hopelessness. Antisocial or hostile behavior is much more common in individuals with opioid dependence than in the general population. Doctors have found that a history of behavior disorder in childhood or adolescence may be a significant risk factor for substance-related disorders, especially opioid dependence.

Opioid abuse is repeated use of an opioid such as heroin or morphine. The person may not be addicted in the sense of a person with opioid dependence—their life does not necessarily revolve around getting the drug—but an abuser does have physical, psychological, social, and legal problems as a result of drug use.

Abuse can be diagnosed when, as a result of heroin use, the patient is unable to attend school or work, cannot perform satisfactorily in a job or at school on multiple occasions, and neglects duties at home or related to family. The abuser will use the substance in dangerous situations (driving a car, for example), may have repeated legal problems (such as arrests for disorderly conduct that are related to substance abuse), and will not stop even after conflicts with loved ones over the effects of the drug on the abuser's personality and life.

People who abuse opioids—"recreational users"—typically use these substances much less frequently than do those with dependence. They may not develop a significant tolerance to the drug or suffer serious symptoms of withdrawal when they stop taking it. When problems related to opioid use are accompanied by evidence of tolerance, withdrawal, or compulsive behavior related to the use of opioids, the doctor should consider a diagnosis of opioid dependence rather than opioid abuse.

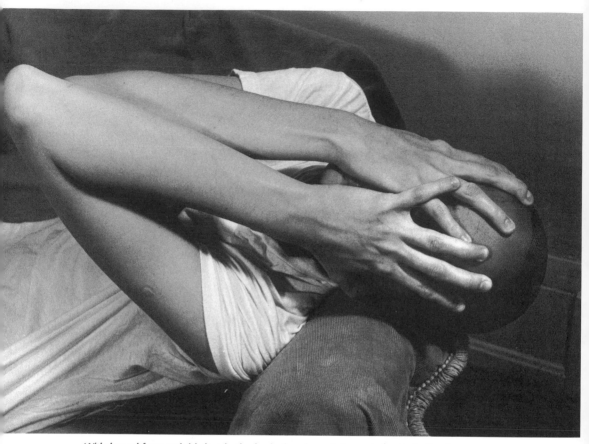

Withdrawal from opioids has both physical and mental symptoms, including fever, nausea, depression, muscle aches, insomnia, and increased sensitivity to pain.

OPIOID INTOXICATION AND WITHDRAWAL

In Chapter 3, the immediate effect of heroin use (the "high," or intoxication) and the effects of discontinuing use of the drug (withdrawal) were discussed briefly. Because these affect the mind as well as the body, they are considered by doctors to be among the psychological effects of the drug.

There are significant behavioral or psychological changes seen in opioid intoxication. These may initially include an elated mood, followed by apathy, depression or anxiety, and psychomotor agitation or retardation (markedly speeded or slowed muscular activity that is associated with mental functioning). Impaired judgment or impaired social or occupational functioning may also develop during, or shortly after, use of an opioid like heroin.

Doctors and clinicians can identify heroin intoxication through several physical signs. The pupils of the eyes are very tiny when a person has taken heroin (unless there has been a severe overdose, in which case a lack of oxygen may cause the pupils of the eyes to dilate), and one or more of the following signs are present: drowsiness (this is known as being "on the nod"), slurred speech, and impairment in attention or memory. Individuals with opioid intoxication may not pay attention to their surroundings, to the point of ignoring potentially harmful situations. The clinician must be certain that these symptoms are not a result of a preexisting medical condition or caused by prescription medication for a health problem.

The scope of the behavioral and physiological changes that result from opioid use depends on the size of the dose as well as characteristics of the individual using the substance (such as tolerance, rate of absorption, and frequency of use). Symptoms of opioid intoxication usually last for several hours. Severe intoxication following an opioid overdose can lead to respiratory depression, unconsciousness, coma, and death.

According to the *DSM-IV*, the essential feature of opioid withdrawal is the presence of withdrawal symptoms after a person who has been a heavy user of a drug such as heroin for an extended time stops taking the drug. In most individuals, withdrawal symptoms occur within 6 to 24 hours after the last dose. Acute withdrawal symptoms for heroin usually peak within one to three days and gradually subside over a period of five to seven days. These symptoms may include depression or anxiety, nausea or vomiting, muscle aches, watery eyes or runny nose, increased sensitivity to pain, widening of the pupils, goosebumps, sweating and fever, and diarrhea. Other symptoms last longer, for weeks or even months, but are less acute: depression, insomnia (inability to sleep), and craving for the drug.

The *DSM-IV* says that three or more of the symptoms listed above must be present for a doctor to diagnose opioid withdrawal. Clinicians must also be careful not to diagnose opioid withdrawal if the symptoms are caused by a general medical condition or another mental disorder.

OTHER OPIOID-INDUCED DISORDERS

There are a number of psychological problems that can occur when a

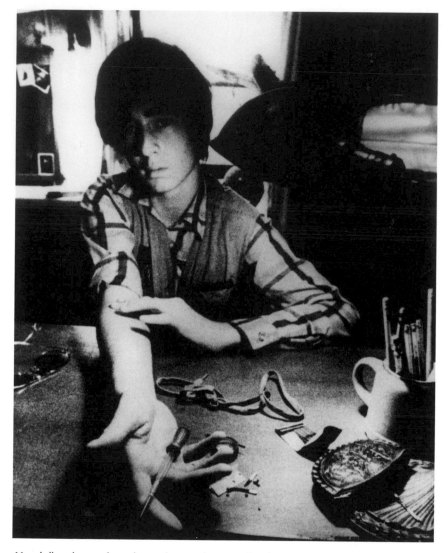

Mood disorders such as depression can be caused or intensified by abuse of opioids.

person uses a drug such as heroin. These include delirium, psychotic disorder, mood swings, sleep disorders, and sexual dysfunction. In most cases, these disorders can occur either during the drug-induced "high" or during the period of withdrawal when a user has stopped taking the drug. Although the symptoms of these disorders are often seen as a part of opioid intoxication or opioid withdrawal, they may be severe enough to warrant separate clinical attention and treatment.

INTOXICATION-DELIRIUM DISORDER

The *DSM-IV* defines delirium as a disturbance of consciousness and the thought process, characterized by:

> . . . a reduced clarity of awareness of the environment. The ability to focus, sustain, or shift attention is impaired. Questions must be repeated because the individual's attention wanders. . . . The person is easily distracted by irrelevant stimuli. Because of these problems, it may be difficult (or impossible) to engage the person in conversation.

A person suffering from delirium often has problems with memory loss (especially recent events), feels disorientated, and may use language incorrectly when speaking. Memory loss can be tested by asking the person to remember several unrelated objects and then to repeat them after a few minutes of distraction. Disorientation includes problems with perception of both time and place. The person may think it is morning when it is actually the middle of the night, believe that events that happened years in the past are occurring in the immediate present, or think they are at home when they are actually in a hospital. Language disturbance may include dysnomia (an impaired ability to name objects), dysgraphia (impaired ability to write), rambling or incoherent speech, and unpredictable conversation swings from subject to subject.

Some people suffering from dementia may have perceptual disturbances, such as hallucinations, illusions, or misinterpretations. The *DSM-IV* gives the examples of mistaking a door banging for a gunshot (misinterpretation), thinking that the folds of blankets on a bed are a living, moving entity (illusion), or "seeing" people or things that are not actually there (hallucination). Although most perceptual disturbances are visual, other senses can be affected as well. The person suffering from dementia often believes strongly that these perceptual disturbances are real and will react accordingly. These disturbances may come and go during the course of a day.

Delirium may cause emotional disturbances such as anxiety, fear, depression, irritability, anger, euphoria, and apathy. It is possible that the person suffering from this disorder may shift rapidly and unpredictably from one emotional state to another, according to the *DSM-IV*.

Use of heroin and other opioids can result in delirium both along with the intoxicating effects of the drug and during withdrawal. Delirium that occurs during intoxication usually only develops after the drug "high" is sustained for several days. Usually, the delirium ends when the intoxication does. Delirium associated with withdrawal develops as the levels of the drug are reduced in a long-term user's body. The symptoms of this delirium may last from a few hours to several weeks.

*PSYCHOTIC DISORDER

Psychotic disorder is characterized by powerful hallucinations or delusions. It is different from dementia in that persons with dementia have periods of lucidity in which they realize that their hallucinations are not real; this is not the case with persons suffering from psychotic disorder.

Psychotic disorder can occur in association with the intoxicating state caused by heroin or along with the symptoms of withdrawal. With heroin or another opioid, the most common delusion is a belief that the user is being persecuted. Hallucinations may include distortion of body image or misperception of people's faces. In addition, users may hallucinate that bugs are crawling in or under their skin, and this can lead to physical damage from extensive scratching.

Psychotic disorder caused by substance abuse does not always end promptly when the drug is removed. The psychiatric effects of the drug can persist for two to four weeks in some cases, depending on the drug user's history and the method of treatment. Psychotic disorder can also occur during withdrawal even if there were no signs of the disorder when the person was taking the drug.

When diagnosing psychotic disorder in a heroin abuser, the doctor should specify the disorder by indicating if delusions (such as the feeling of being persecuted or of having power) or hallucinations (for example, imagining that bugs are crawling on one's skin) are the predominant symptom. The clinician should also note whether the psychotic disorder's onset occurred during intoxication or during withdrawal.

*MOOD DISORDER

The essential feature of a substance-induced mood disorder is a persistent disturbance in mood that is judged to be caused directly by the drug, rather than by some other factor such as a preexisting medical condition. The disorder may result in depression, irritability, or an elevated, expansive mood.

Mood disorders are a common side effect of drug abuse; this may be

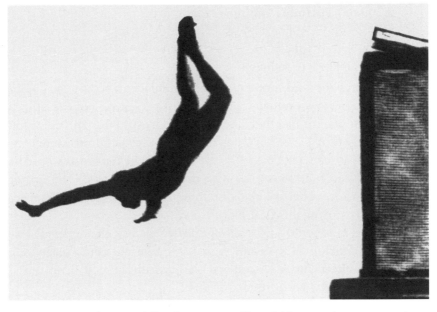

In extreme cases, the mental disturbances caused by opioid use can become so unpleasant or severe that the user may attempt suicide.

because of mood swings that occur when the user comes down from the artificial "high" caused by the drug. The *DSM-IV* lists four types of mood episodes—major depressive, manic, hypomanic, and mixed—and explains them as follows:

- A **major depressive episode** is characterized by at least two weeks of depressed mood or loss of interest in school, work, or family activities, accompanied by additional symptoms of depression (i.e., change in appetite, sleep problems, decreased energy, or difficulty making decisions).

- A **manic episode** is defined by a period of an abnormally and persistently elevated, expansive, or irritable mood lasting at least one week. Other symptoms include inflated self-esteem, decreased need for sleep, an increase in creative thinking, and distractibility.

- A **hypomanic episode** is similar to a manic episode, except that the period of elevated mood does not last as long and the elevated mood is not as high.

- A **mixed episode** combines the symptoms of a manic episode and a major depressive episode during a brief period. The individual experiences rapidly alternating moods, from euphoria to sadness.

A substance-induced mood disorder can be identified by the doctor according to the predominant episode that is presented. For example, if a psychiatrist determined that a heroin user was suffering from a mood disorder caused by his or her drug abuse and the symptoms were consistent with those of a major depressive episode, the diagnosis would be "opioid-induced mood disorder with depressive features." The doctor would also note whether the development of the mood disorder occurred first during intoxication or the withdrawal period.

Diagnosis of mood disorder should not be made if the person is suffering from delirium. The doctor must also be careful not to diagnose a substance-induced mood disorder if the patient suffered from mood swings not caused by drug use in the past.

✳ SLEEP DISORDER

Problems with sleep patterns are another psychological problem caused by heroin abuse. If the disturbance in the sleep-wake cycle has a very strong effect on the person's ability to function and is judged to be the direct result of substance abuse, then opioid-induced sleep disorder may be diagnosed.

In the short term, opioids such as heroin cause an increase in sleepiness, and the user falls into a deeper sleep than he or she otherwise might. However, as tolerance to the drug increases, so does tolerance to heroin's sedative effects, and the user may experience periods of insomnia. The main feature of insomnia is difficulty initiating or maintaining sleep over a one-month period, and this difficulty causes distress or impairment at home, at work, or in social situations. People with insomnia often have the combination of trouble falling asleep and intermittent periods of wakefulness when they do get to sleep, and their sleep is often nonrestorative—that is, they do not feel rested when they awaken.

When a person is going through opioid withdrawal, complaints of hypersomnia are common. Hypersomnia is the opposite of insomnia. It is characterized by excessive sleepiness for at least one month, including either lengthy sleep episodes or frequent periods of sleep that occur during the day. As with insomnia, the excessive sleepiness causes distress or impairment at home, at work, or in social situations.

Parasomnias are another type of substance-induced sleep disorder. According to the *DSM-IV*, these are characterized by "complaints of unusual behavior during sleep." The parasomnias include nightmares, sleep terror disorder (being awakened from sleep abruptly in a state of great fear), and sleepwalking.

It is also possible for a person with an opioid-induced sleep disorder to suffer from symptoms of more than one of these specific disorders— for example, insomnia combined with sleep terror—without one form being prevalent. In this case, a mixed-type sleep disorder would be diagnosed.

✳ SEXUAL DYSFUNCTION

Use of heroin or other drugs can affect interpersonal relationships, and sexual dysfunction is common. The dysfunction may involve a lack of desire for sex, difficulty becoming sexually aroused, an inability to achieve orgasm, or pain associated with sexual intercourse.

The *DSM-IV* notes that opioid-induced sexual dysfunctions usually begin during intoxication. Men and women who use heroin are equally likely to suffer from sexual dysfunction.

■　　　　　■　　　　　■

Obviously, there are many psychological problems associated with heroin use, in addition to the physical problems that the drug causes. Both the physical and psychological components of the drug may have an effect on addiction, as described in the next chapter.

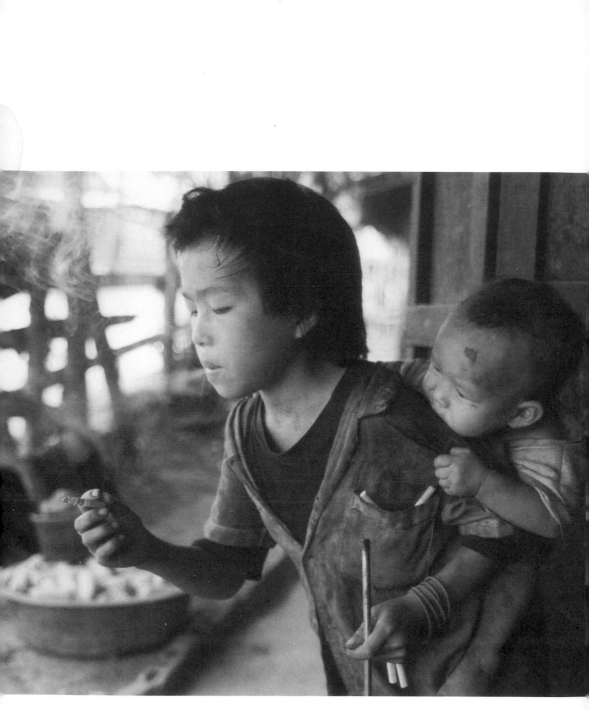

A 12-year-old boy in Thailand smokes a cigarette and holds his heroin pipe. Heroin use is spreading among the hill tribes of Thailand as their lifestyle becomes more modernized. A large percentage of the world's opium poppies are grown in Thailand, making opiate drugs more easily available there.

5

THE CAUSES OF
HEROIN ADDICTION

In November 1997, a panel convened by the National Institutes of Health declared that heroin addiction should be treated as a disease. "Opiate addiction is a mental disorder and basically is a brain-related disease," Lewis Judd, chairman of the Department of Psychiatry at the University of California, San Diego, and head of the panel, told *USA Today*. "It is not a weakness of the will or a moral issue."

Most health care professionals agree that addiction may best be understood as a form of disease. But what does this mean? Disease is a condition in a living organism that impairs its normal function and can be recognized by symptoms that follow a common course. This would seem to be an accurate description of heroin addiction, from what we've learned in earlier chapters. However, most diseases occur because of a virus or because of defective genetic material. People don't choose to get tuberculosis or muscular dystrophy, but they can choose not to take drugs. Therefore, doctors say that use of an addictive drug is not a disease, but addiction to the drug is because addiction is involuntary.

Over the years heroin has been one of the most studied of addictive drugs, because the drug affects so many aspects of an addict's life. The effects of heroin have been studied by sociologists, doctors, and psychologists, who are all trying to learn more. As a result, there have been multiple ideas about how and why some people become heroin addicts.

PHYSIOLOGICAL FACTORS

Some doctors believe that addiction to heroin is purely a physical reaction of chemicals in the brain and central nervous system. In the 1970s scientists first began to understand how and why opioids like heroin affect the human brain. They discovered that when the drug enters a user's bloodstream, opioid molecules attach themselves to certain parts of the brain, called receptors, as well as to the neurons of the central nervous system. The binding together of the opioid and the receptor produces an electrical charge in the nervous system that causes feelings of pleasure.

Why would the human brain and nervous system have receptors that allow a drug like heroin to affect their function? This question led scientists to the discovery of a natural substance produced by the body, which they named endorphins (Greek for "morphine inside us"). Endorphins are protein compounds that are produced in the human pituitary gland and released into the bloodstream constantly, often in response to outside stimuli. These proteins are neurotransmitters, meaning that they affect the neurological messages from the nervous system to the brain and help regulate responses to internal and external events such as stress, pain, or excitement. Endorphins have been called "the brain's own natural painkillers" and may contribute to euphoric feelings such as the "runner's high" experienced after prolonged exercise.

Scientists discovered that heroin and other opioids mimic the effects of endorphins on the human brain, linking to the receptors to stimulate feelings of pleasure. However, the human neurological system is very complicated and very delicate, and drugs overload the system with false messages. When heroin or another opioid is injected into the body, the level of these pleasure-causing opioids is much greater than the human body's endorphin system is supposed to receive. One theory of addiction says that this overload of opiate-simulated endorphins leads the brain to change how it works and to become dependent on the drug. Scientists believe that the body is tricked by the high level of artificial endorphins that result from taking the drug and stops producing natural endorphins. When the drug's effects wear off but the body no longer produces endorphins, withdrawal symptoms result. The user enters a vicious cycle in which more and more external substances are needed to produce the endorphins that help the body cope with stress and pain.

There are other, related physiological theories of addiction. Some doctors have speculated that heroin addicts are born with faulty endorphin systems, and other researchers have claimed that addicts developed endorphin problems before using opioids. An old idea that is it possible to be "addicted to pleasure" has also been revived. With the discovery of receptor sites—certain areas of the brain devoted solely to pleasure— some doctors believe that when heroin overwhelms the neurological

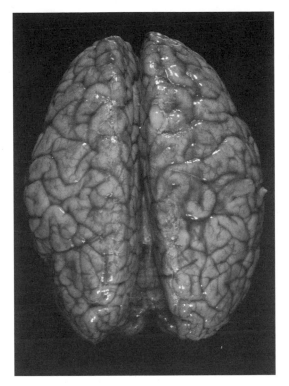

Heroin affects the brain by mimicking neurotransmitters called endorphins, which cause euphoria and reduce pain.

system, the feelings of pleasure are so strong that the brain can no longer focus on the healthy stimuli of everyday life—love, good food, or praise—but demands focus on the effects of the heroin.

It is clear that heroin use changes how the brain processes feelings and experiences long after drug use stops. Researchers and doctors who believe that heroin addiction is solely physiological believe that there may be an endorphin, or a substitute for the drug, that can be introduced to an addict's system to cure addiction.

PSYCHOLOGICAL AND ENVIRONMENTAL FACTORS

For many years, popular opinion considered heroin addiction to be immoral behavior by deviant or criminal personalities. Early studies that evaluated addicts in prisons or on the streets indicated that heroin users exhibited sociopathic behavior. A sociopath is considered to be lacking the instincts that are essential for forming caring human relationships. These studies reinforced the stereotypes of the addict as a bad person.

In the 1930s and '40s, psychiatrists began evaluating heroin addicts at

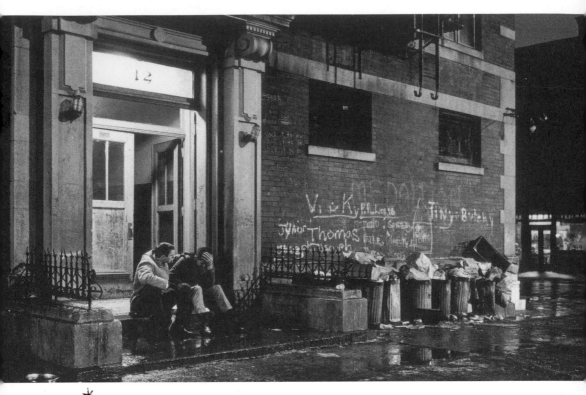

Environmental factors may also contribute to heroin addiction; people living in inner cities, especially in neighborhoods with large numbers of addicts, may be more likely to use heroin themselves.

the Addiction Research Center in Kentucky, expecting to learn about the criminal mind. The researchers were unable to determine a common element that would suggest tendencies to crime in heroin users; instead, they found a broad spectrum of personality features.

By the 1960s, new characterizations of the addict had begun to replace the older stereotypes. Some theorists now believe that addictions are caused by psychological drives, and they often refer to the "addictive personality" to describe people with overpowering psychological obsessions with using drugs, food, relationships, or gambling to change the way they feel.

Although there is no "criminal" personality linked to heroin abuse, research has shown that some types of people are more likely to become addicted to drugs. A young adult with low self-esteem, for example, may say, "Why shouldn't I take drugs? I'm a loser anyway." The drug intoxication may temporarily lift feelings of depression. Drug use may also be a way to fit into the crowd, and peer pressure is often an important reason a young person begins to use drugs. Most young addicts start with legal drugs (although these are illegal for minors to use) like nicotine and alcohol, then "graduate" to marijuana and then to something stronger like cocaine or heroin. The young drug user often gets the substances from friends and uses them to feel part of the group.

Another theory of drug addiction proposes that, because of low self-esteem, some people become addicted in order to slowly commit suicide. Long-term addicts often express self-hatred and believe that their continued use of the drug is self-destructive. However, few people begin taking drugs with a conscious desire to kill themselves, so those feelings are probably unconscious and develop during the course of addiction.

Environmental factors can also affect the rate of addiction. In inner-city neighborhoods, drugs may be easier to get than in rural communities, and as a result drug addiction is more common. However, there are drug problems in every community. Young adults living in nice suburban neighborhoods often have money and time on their hands—a feeling that there is "nothing to do." These teens may opt to use the drugs that are available in the cities.

Also, circumstances may help users to feel that it is all right to use drugs. One of the most important studies of heroin addiction focused on U.S. servicemen in Vietnam. Heroin was cheap and easy to get during the war, and many soldiers became addicted while they were in Vietnam. Military treatment programs were not successful in preventing relapses among patients who returned to active duty in the field. However, when the soldiers returned to the United States, only about 5 percent of the addicts continued to be chronic heroin users. Researchers interpreted this remarkable statistic to mean that setting is a very important part of addiction.

■　　　　■　　　　■

While there is no shortage of theories on the causes of heroin addiction, the truth is that addiction is probably a combination of psychological, physiological, and environmental factors. The next chapter will show how both the physical and psychological effects of heroin are treated in an attempt to break the cycle of dependence caused by the drug addiction.

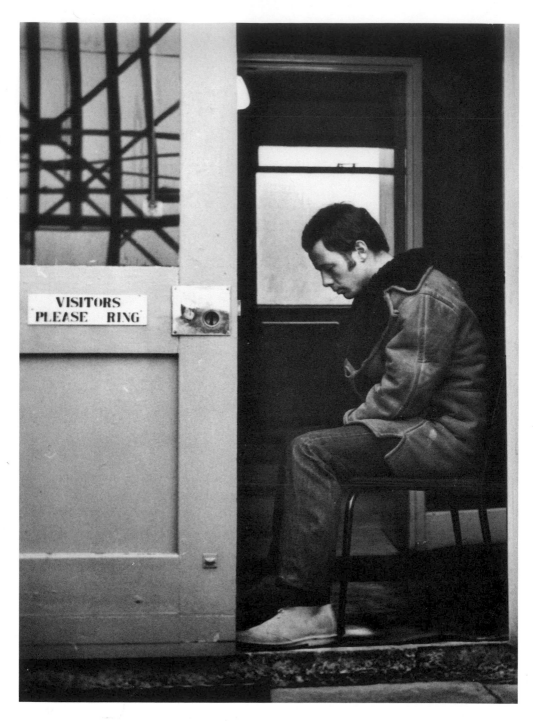

An addict sits at the entrance to a drug treatment center in Portsmouth, England, while he makes sure he truly wants to quit. Heroin is one of the most addictive drugs and one of the hardest to "kick."

6

TREATMENT OF HEROIN ADDICTION

Because the physical and psychological problems discussed in Chapters 3 and 4 have a direct relationship to heroin use, doctors must break the drug addiction in order to treat these disorders. There are several forms of treatment used to end a person's physical and psychological dependence on heroin. Although drug detoxification—the term used for removing drug toxins from an addict's system—is often the route into treatment, many who begin the process do not complete it, and many who complete it do not go on to more definitive treatment. Some enter only to lower their level of dependence and to have an easier time supporting their habit, but others, especially younger addicted persons who have not yet frequently relapsed, fully believe that detoxification is all that is necessary to kick the habit completely.

Physicians are now focusing on approaches that they feel are most likely to keep the patient in treatment for both detoxification and the next stage. The ideal detoxification method would be relatively short, inexpensive, and painless; could be done on an outpatient basis; and would leave the patient with a desire to seek longer-term help. Although none of the techniques reviewed here is perfect, it appears that society is closing in on more effective methods of drug treatment. Compared to 50 years ago, patients today can be detoxified with little discomfort and in a much shorter period of time.

EVALUATION AND DIAGNOSIS

A doctor's initial evaluation determines the best way to begin treating the addiction to heroin. Once the person is in treatment, a more complete mental and physical assessment is used to devise an individual treatment plan. The medical interview is key to determining the most effective form of treatment by helping the physician learn these things about the patient:

- Drug history: Has the patient used drugs in the past, or is there a drug problem now? If so, how long has the drug been used, and how frequently? When was the drug last used? How was the drug taken (injection, sniffing, etc.)? What was the size of the dose? Why was it taken (to get high, to relieve depression, etc.)? Any previous treatment will also be noted, including where treatment took place, what type of treatment was involved, and the outcome.
- Medical history: The doctor will give special attention to the possible medical complications of drug abuse, especially illnesses that may complicate withdrawal or that have been ignored because of the patient's chaotic lifestyle.
- Social functioning: The physician will ask about the patient's living arrangements, marital status, sexual orientation, employment and/or educational status, education, psychological state, history of drug or alcohol problems (if any), friends, recreational activities, and if the patient has had problems with the law.
- Psychological status: In addition to factors that could complicate withdrawal, such as severe depression or suicidal tendencies, the physician can look for conditions for which special treatments exist. It is helpful, though difficult, to see whether psychiatric conditions came before or after the drug abuse. Opioids may ease some psychiatric conditions, and withdrawal can lead to sudden appearance or worsening of psychotic symptoms.
- Physical condition: The patient will take a number of physical tests, including a blood chemistry profile, a test for HIV, an electrocardiogram to test the strength of the patient's heart, a chest X-ray, skin tests, and other tests the doctor feels are necessary.

DETOXIFICATION

Detoxification, or "detox", is the process of removing the opiates from the addict's system. Because addiction to opiates produces physical dependence, detoxification will often have at least some of the side effects expected in withdrawal, especially if the addict is heavily addicted or is attempting to detoxify "cold turkey"—that is, without the aid of any other medications or therapy.

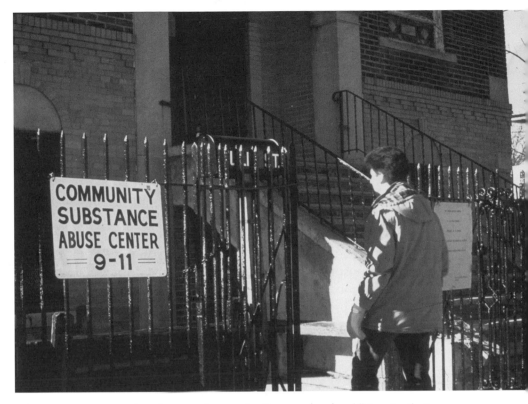

A man enters a community substance abuse center. For some heroin addicts, outpatient treatment such as this center provides will be enough to help them kick the habit.

Until the 1960s, detoxification was the only method available to addicts seeking treatment; it was believed to be the essential part of successful treatment for addiction. Most often, the process involved a gradual reduction of the amount of opiates the addict received each day until the physical dependence had been overcome and the addict no longer needed the drug. Sometimes methadone was substituted for morphine or heroin, because the withdrawal from methadone is less painful and less severe. At the end of the detoxification process, the addicts were released from the clinics with no further treatment; most of them, unfortunately, relapsed into addiction. This often began a cycle of addiction and detoxification that could last for years, because even after the physical dependence on opiates is ended, the cravings for the drug may recur long after detoxification.

Today, detoxification is seen as the beginning of an addict's treatment. An addict who checks into a treatment clinic for "residential" detoxification typically receives prescribed amounts of other drugs (usually methadone, although research has shown that the hypertension drug Clonidine, which is not an opiate, may also ease withdrawal symptoms) to take as a substitute for the opiates on which he or she is dependent. Because the symptoms of withdrawal from methadone are milder than those of morphine or heroin, and since methadone remains active in the body longer, an addict can function at a fairly normal level and not suffer from drug cravings for up to a day before needing the next, smaller dose. Heroin dependency can usually be ended in this manner in one to three weeks. Addicts with less severe dependencies may be treated as outpatients, in "community" detoxification settings, if they are deemed sufficiently motivated. Of course, the addict must follow the program of treatment through to the end and must stop using the drugs that caused the dependence as soon as the treatment program begins. It is estimated that only 15 percent of the addicts who begin detoxification complete the regimen and go on to further stages of recovery.

Recently, a controversial new detoxification program has been developed. The new process is intended to complete the detoxification process entirely within one day and involves the use of an opiate antagonist (naloxene or naltrexone) while the patient is under general anesthesia. The antagonist is a drug that is stronger than an opioid and attaches to the same receptors in the brain that an opiate would, although it does not have the same effect as a painkiller and relaxant. The opiate antagonist basically pushes the opioids out of its way as it links to the receptor sites, and thus prevents the heroin or morphine from affecting the patient. It is administered either intravenously (naloxene) or orally (naltrexone) and accelerates the process of withdrawal. In this type of rapid detoxification, which takes between four and six hours, the patient experiences severe withdrawal symptoms while remaining under anesthesia. Normally a breathing tube is inserted in the windpipe to protect against choking, which can occur if the patient vomits.

Supporters of the new technique claim that the rapid detoxification benefits patients who are ready to go on to full recovery and who may have difficulty with traditional detoxification procedures. They also point out that this method does not induce any dependence on anoth-

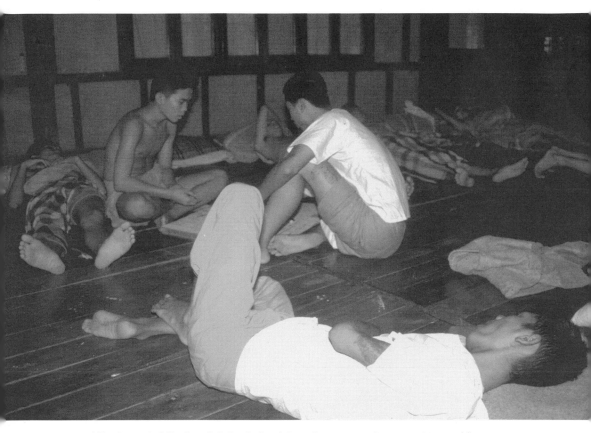

Addicts in a rehabilitation clinic in Thailand, in various stages of recovery. Many addicts need residential treatment so that they can detoxify in a drug-free, controlled environment.

er substance (such as methadone) in the process of ending the original opiate dependence. Critics argue that the method has not been tested thoroughly enough to be pronounced safe (there are only six published studies with a total of 63 cases currently available) and that if it is touted as an "easy cure" for addiction, it will draw attention away from the need for addicts to go on to further therapy and rehabilitation once the drugs are out of their bodies. They also question whether the rate of relapse will increase with the new technique, because the addict does not feel any of the symptoms of withdrawal and thus does not view the withdrawal process as a deterrent to another cycle of addiction. Currently, there are no set guidelines for all clinics which offer this service, although it has been made available on a trial basis in the United States and Canada. Most clinics which offer the technique offer further rehabilitative treatment and therapy to their patients in the weeks or months following their detoxification.

METHADONE MAINTENANCE

Methadone is a synthetic opioid that was developed in Germany during World War II as a painkiller that could be substituted for morphine. Since the 1960s, methadone has been used to treat long-term addicts whose body chemistries have changed to require a constant supply of

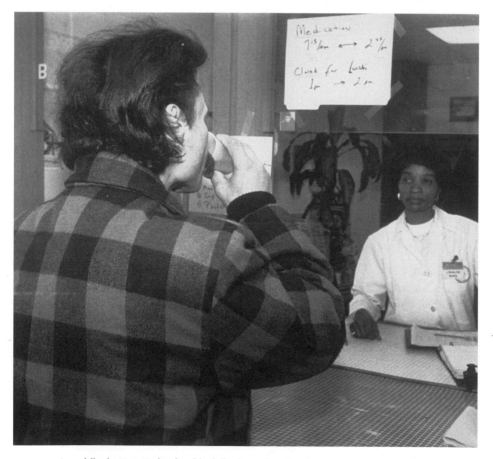

An addict in New York takes his daily dose of methadone as a nurse supervises. Methadone maintenance can sometimes help a long-term or heavy addict to regain control of his or her life.

opioids. The effects of methadone are less intense than the effects of heroin, but the drug remains in the user's system longer.

When properly prescribed, methadone does not have the intoxicating effects of heroin and suppresses the symptoms of heroin withdrawal. Methadone does not seem to interfere with everyday activities, such as reading a newspaper or driving a car. However, it is not always simple to prescribe the proper dose. If a patient on methadone maintenance becomes intoxicated, he or she is taking too much of the drug.

When a patient has been taking narcotics for medical purposes, the medicinal dose can be converted into an equivalent dose of methadone very simply. However, when a patient has been using illegal drugs, the picture is very different. The amount of heroin sold in a bag on the street can vary from city to city, from dealer to dealer, and even from day to day. The quality and purity of heroin sold on the street has increased greatly in the past few years. Under these circumstances, the physician must guess at the initial dose. The initial dose of methadone must be high enough to subdue withdrawal symptoms adequately but, because large amounts of methadone can be fatal, low enough that if the

EARLY ATTEMPTS AT TREATMENT

By 1910, several physicians had experimented with treatments for heroin addiction. Drs. Alexander Lambert and Charles B. Towns touted their popular cure as the most "advanced, effective, and compassionate" cure for addiction to opiates. The cure consisted of a seven-day regimen, including a five-day purge of heroin from the addict's system with doses of belladonna, a natural tranquilizer that comes from a poisonous plant and has been used as an herbal medicine since ancient times. The chemicals in belladonna were believed to help remove opiates from the stomach and intestinal tract. If these opiate toxins could be removed from the body, the theory went, the addiction would end. Another popular "cure" was offered by private hospitals, called sanitariums, which confined patients as they suffered through the agony of withdrawal. These clinics claimed their methods were successful 90 percent of the time. However, most of the hard-core addicts who tried these cures returned to opiate use within six months.

patient's tolerance is not as high as the doctor believes, the treatment will not be detrimental to the patient's health.

A person who has been given methadone for the first time will be kept under observation so the effect of the dose can be judged. The methadone should suppress withdrawal symptoms within 30 to 60 minutes; if it does not, an additional dose can be given. If withdrawal symptoms are not present, the patient should be observed for drowsiness or slowed breathing.

Studies of methadone maintenance programs show that one-third of patients improve, one-third vacillate between good and bad performance, and one-third show no change from a lifestyle centered on drugs and crime. Although this response rate is less than perfect, before methadone there was no way to effect the positive outcome of the one-third of patients who do well or the successful periods of treatment for the one-third who go back and forth. Methadone, for most opioid-dependent persons, is not a cure, but substantial benefits result from its proper use. For example, research indicates that methadone maintenance programs have prevented many opiate-injecting persons from getting HIV, and there is substantial evidence that needle use and sharing are lessened when addicted persons enter methadone programs.

LENGTH OF TREATMENT

The symptoms of opioid withdrawal (rather than the patient's complaints alone) should determine the course of treatment. However, certain signs, such as pupillary dilatation, may be modified by the dosage of methadone even when the patient is undermedicated. After the patient is stabilized, the dose is gradually withdrawn. In general, inpatient withdrawal takes 5 to 10 days, whereas outpatient withdrawal may take longer to ensure that the patient does not end the treatment before it is completed.

Although insomnia, fatigue, and anxiety can linger for weeks or months, acute withdrawal is considered over if there are no signs of acute opioid withdrawal—muscle cramps, nausea, hallucinations, and convulsions—48 hours after the last dose of methadone. A mild rebound in withdrawal symptoms has been noted after the last dose of methadone, but this generally recedes over the next few weeks.

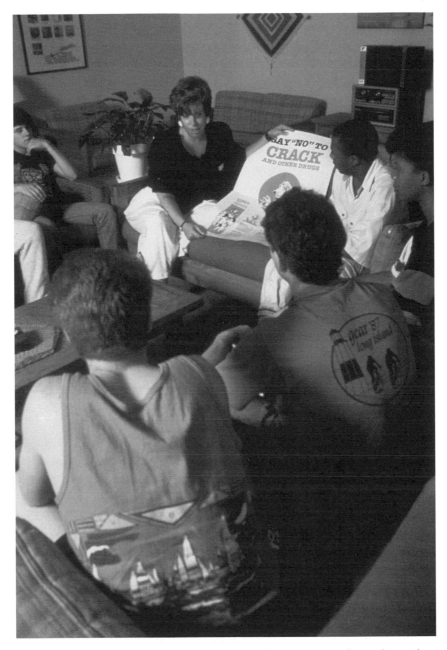

Teens in a counseling center discuss the effects of drug abuse. Counseling or therapy is a major part of most recovery programs.

PROBLEMS ASSOCIATED WITH DETOXIFICATION

In addition to the difficulties of withdrawal, addicts attempting to end their dependence on heroin or another opiate occasionally suffer from other physical problems.

Seizures do not usually result from opioid withdrawal or intoxication. A seizure, therefore, usually signifies that there may be undiagnosed withdrawal from another sedative, or tranquilizing, drug (such as alcohol, barbiturate, or benzodiazepines); that another medical condition exists (such as a head injury or epilepsy); or that the seizure may be faked.

A mixed addiction, including sedative dependence in addition to heroin addiction, can lead to seizures, hypothermia (dangerously lowered body temperatures), and even death. If a mixed addiction is present, the patient is often placed on methadone, withdrawn from the sedative gradually, and then withdrawn from the methadone. With-

ADDICTION AND PREGNANCY

When pregnancy is complicated by heroin addiction, the patient and her physician are faced with making the best of some difficult choices. The best circumstance would be for the patient to abstain totally from drugs, legal or illegal, during the pregnancy. Unfortunately, this is often not likely to occur. On an outpatient drug-free regimen, many patients go in and out of heroin use, subjecting the fetus to periods of intoxication and withdrawal and increasing the risk of stillbirth, premature birth, and birth defects.

The drug's effects are compounded by the pregnant patient's lifestyle, poor prenatal care, inadequate diet, and drug additives. Residential placement to ensure a drug-free status is usually resisted by the mother or hard to find. Narcotic antagonists, drugs that can help withdrawal, have not yet been approved for maintenance during pregnancy. Methadone maintenance at the lowest dose possible is left as the least undesirable option for most such patients. The infant will be born addicted and may need to be withdrawn from the drug but otherwise should not have problems if there has been adequate obstetrical care during the pregnancy.

drawal from stimulant-type drugs poses less of a physical hazard than withdrawal from opioids, but it can be associated with severe depression and even suicide.

Although vomiting can be a symptom of withdrawal, it can occur with no relation to the degree of physical abstinence and in spite of all kinds of supporting measures, including reuse of opioids. Vomiting can usually be treated with antinausea drugs.

When an addict trying to kick heroin has other serious medical problems, withdrawal from the drug should be very gradual. With certain illnesses, including heart and kidney disease, the patient should be maintained on methadone until he or she is stable enough to go through withdrawal.

THERAPY AND COUNSELING

The final step in successful heroin addiction treatment is therapy. Over the years, various forms of therapy have been proposed and tried, with the goal of helping the addict become a fully functional member of society, encouraging him or her to stay sober and not relapse. Twelve-step programs, psychotherapy, and stays in therapeutic communities have all filled this need.

For the most serious addict, the therapeutic community probably offers the best recovery strategy. In a therapeutic community, recovering addicts live for six to 24 months in a controlled setting where no drugs of any kind are permitted. The programs are often run by former addicts in conjunction with psychologists. While they live in the treatment center, addicts may receive vocational and educational training to help them re-enter the outside world more effectively. While some 75 percent of residents leave the therapeutic communities within the first six months, those who stay for the full course of treatment have a 90 percent success rate in staying drug-free.

For slightly less severely addicted patients, psychological counseling in a non-residential setting is another option. The therapist offers the addict a safe space to come to terms with addiction and express fears, anxiety, or pain. Sometimes addicts meet for group counseling, which allows them to support one another on the road to recovery.

Twelve-step programs such as Narcotics Anonymous work in much the same way. Typically self-help groups made up entirely of recovering addicts, they meet regularly to share support, advice, and consultation. The programs aim to help addicts find a sense of control by teaching them to take their recovery "one day at a time" and giving them a safety net of people they can turn to if they fear they will relapse.

POSITIVE BENEFITS OF TREATMENT

In addition to helping a user become drug free, treatment programs have other effects. These include reducing demand for illegal drugs, changing users' personal values, developing educational and vocational capabilities, improving users' overall health, and reducing fetal exposure to drugs. Because many addicted persons commit crimes to get money for illegal opioids, an indirect effect of legal methadone is to reduce or eliminate associated crime.

AFTER TREATMENT IS COMPLETE

Despite the power that heroin holds over an addict, it is possible to recover from addiction to the drug. Any established treatment facility can point to "graduates" who have been able to change their lives and give up the drug, and nearly every day in the news there is another story of a former addict gone straight who is now willing to discuss what it took to "kick the habit." It is estimated that about half the people who complete long-term residential treatment programs can remain drug free indefinitely.

Overcoming heroin addiction requires a commitment to a changed lifestyle. After a program of treatment and therapy is complete, the former user should surround himself or herself with friends who do not use opioids and who will support efforts to avoid the drug. One slip could plunge the former addict back into the cycle of dependence.

■　　　　　■　　　　　■

Although some patients see detoxification as the only treatment necessary for stable abstinence, most patients and clinicians view it as only the first step in the long process of remaining off illicit drugs. Regardless of the treatment program, many users believe they can return to occasional use. However, these users are quickly "hooked" again and return to their addictive patterns of behavior. Much like a recovering alcoholic, who knows that the next drink could start the cycle all over again, a heroin addict must learn to accept that not using the drug for several months or years is not a sign that he or she is "cured." Former users must continue to lead a drug-free lifestyle to maintain control of their lives.

Success, therefore, is a function not just of how painless the procedure is but of the number of patients retained and the likelihood they will go on to longer-term treatment. Whatever method is chosen, there must be appropriate education and therapy to prepare the patient for this next step.

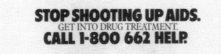

SHARING NEEDLES CAN GET YOU MORE THAN HIGH.

IT CAN GET YOU AIDS.

You can't tell if someone has the AIDS virus just by looking.

You can't tell if needles or works are infected just by looking.

When you shoot drugs and share needles or works you could get AIDS. Even if you think your drug-sharing partners are clean, if the AIDS virus is present, it could be passed to you.

AIDS is not pretty. It's a long, slow, painful way to die. Do the right thing. Get into treatment. It's the best way to make sure you don't shoot up AIDS.

STOP SHOOTING UP AIDS.
GET INTO DRUG TREATMENT.
CALL 1-800 662 HELP.

A Public Service of the National Institute on Drug Abuse, Department of Health and Human Services.

Part of an ad campaign by the National Institute on Drug Abuse, highlighting the health risks of injecting heroin, one of the reasons many addicts decide to quit.

7

MAKING A
COMPLETE RECOVERY

The following excerpt is taken from William S. Burroughs's 1959 novel *Naked Lunch,* which deals with the world of the addict in very graphic terms. Burroughs himself was a heroin addict for 15 years. Here, he discusses his addiction—which he calls "The Sickness"—and the moment when he realizes that he is out of money and out of control, and flies to London to be treated for his drug dependence.

I awoke from The Sickness at the age of forty-five, calm and sane, and in reasonably good health except for a weakened liver and the look of borrowed flesh common to all those who survive The Sickness . . . . The Sickness is drug addiction and I was an addict for fifteen years. When I say addict I mean an addict to junk (generic term for opium and/or derivatives including all synthetics from demerol to palfium). I have used junk in many forms: morphine, heroin, dilaudid, eukodal, pantopon, diocodid, diosane, opium, demerol, dolophine, palfium. . . . I lived in one room in the Native Quarter of Tangier. I had not taken a bath in a year nor changed my clothes or removed them except to stick a needle every hour in the fibrous grey wooden flesh of terminal addiction. I never cleaned or dusted the room. Empty ampoule boxes and garbage piled to the ceiling. Light and water long since turned off for non-payment. I did absolutely nothing. I could look at the end of my shoe for eight hours. I was only roused to action when the hourglass of junk ran out. If a friend came to visit—and they rarely did since who or what was left to visit—I sat there not caring that he had entered my field of vision—a grey screen always blanker and fainter—and not caring when he walked out of it. If he had died on the spot I would have sat there looking at my shoe waiting to go through his pockets. Wouldn't you? Because I never had enough junk— no one ever does. Thirty grains of morphine a day and it was still not enough. And long waits in front of the drugstore. Delay is a rule in the

Most recovering addicts realize that in order to get a job and keep it, they must remain drug free. Many workplaces in the United States now test their applicants and/or employees for drug use.

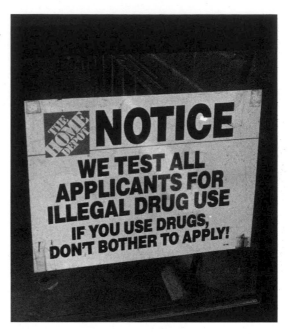

junk business. The Man is never on time. This is no accident. There are no accidents in the junk world. The addict is taught again and again exactly what will happen if he does not score for his junk ration. Get up that money or else. And suddenly my habit began to jump and jump. Forty, sixty grains a day. And still it was not enough. And I could not pay.

I stood there with my last check in hand and realized that it was my last check. I took the next plane for London [and treatment].

OVERCOMING ADDICTION

Detoxification and therapy are only the beginning of a person's recovery from heroin addiction. The recovering addict must make a strong personal commitment to remaining drug free after finishing a program of treatment. Often, a support network of friends and family members must be involved in creating a better environment for recovering addicts, helping them find other ways to relax, enjoy life, and deal with stress. The addict must find ways to change the factors which led to drug abuse in his or her "old" life.

The first step to complete recovery is the addict's decision to make a change. Addicts who go through detoxification treatments without a strong desire to cease their addiction almost always—about 90 percent of the time—relapse once their treatment ends. To stop using heroin permanently, an addict must want to stop and turn his or her life around. Usually this step is the hardest one to take and the most significant in the recovery process. When recovering addicts go through withdrawal, surviving the misery of it and seeing that they had the strength to fight the withdrawal sickness can give them a sense of pride. Not giving in to the craving for heroin becomes an accomplishment for the recovering addict. Each successful fight against the psychological craving for heroin becomes more evidence for the addict of his or her own inner strength.

The change is not limited to simply stopping the use of the drug, however. The addicts' relationships with themselves and with others also must be redefined. For many addicts, their views of authority figures have been extremely negative during the addiction period, and learning to trust that an authority is not always an enemy becomes an important step. Addicts may distrust themselves, feeling that they are not capable of fitting into a normal, drug-free society. Like any time a person has to build up trust, this process takes time, as the addict sees himself or herself living each day drug free and learning how to fit in. In many cases, drug abuse began when the addict was a teenager, stunting the growth and maturing process of the addict's social skills. Addicts in these cases may find that counseling sessions, as well as support from friends and family who are willing to talk with them about their experiences, help them learn to interact with others on a healthy, adult level. Supportive and drug-free peers can also help the recovering addict avoid the feelings of stigma and loneliness which often prompt episodes of drug cravings.

While developing relationships with drug-free friends and family, the addict must also end relationships with active users. Their continued presence in the addict's circle of friends can put destructive pressure on the recovery process. Even if they do not seem to encourage drug use actively, their presence is associated in the addict's mind with using heroin, and this may trigger the conditioned response of drug cravings. Studies have shown that recovering addicts who come into contact with other heroin users during their recovery are much more likely to relapse. This makes recovery especially difficult for someone who is living in a neighborhood with a large number of users. If there is any way to get out of the active-user environment, the recovering addict should take it.

The risk of relapse is always present in the recovering addict's life, but it can be reduced if the person can avoid situations where heroin or other drugs, such as cocaine or marijuana, or even legal substances like alcohol, are frequently used. The addict must learn to say no to offers of other drugs, even though they may seem "less serious" than heroin, because using them can cloud the person's judgment and weaken convictions, making it harder to abstain from heroin use. Recovering heroin addicts are also more likely than other people to develop dependencies on other substances if they start using them, even if they do not return to heroin.

Intimate relationships can be among the most difficult to reform. Although many users feel that drugs are a sexual aid when they first begin to take them, long-term heroin use frequently causes sexual dysfunction and/or disinterest. The partner of a recovering addict must be patient and supportive, helping the addict to cope with fears, insecurities, and difficulties. Sometimes, the process of rebuilding intimacy requires the help of a professional therapist.

Another important part of the return to normal society is employment. Remaining employed is closely linked with remaining drug free in almost all cases, and certainly the ability to remain employed is a sign that rehabilitation is succeeding. Frequently, however, recovering addicts have trouble finding jobs, due to the problems their addiction has caused in the past—lack of skills, poor work records, and periods of unexplained unemployment. Many addicts also find the stresses of the workplace alienating when they begin new jobs. Vocational training as part of treatment can help to alleviate some of these problems, but returning to work remains one of the most problematic steps of recovery.

Doctors also must be aware of a patient's history of heroin abuse when prescribing pain medication. The body of a former addict is often unable to distinguish between the illicit substance and prescribed doses of a legal opiate painkiller like codeine or Dilaudid, and it may return to its former dependent patterns. Whenever possible, recovering addicts should use non-opiate pain therapies, such as acupuncture, massage, or non-opiate medications. If opiates are prescribed, the addict must exercise extreme caution in their use and make sure that there is some supportive person who can monitor his or her intake.

To recover fully, an addict must be able to have fun and relax without using drugs. Finding creative outlets or beginning exercise programs are some of the best ways to do this. This process, called de-addiction, helps

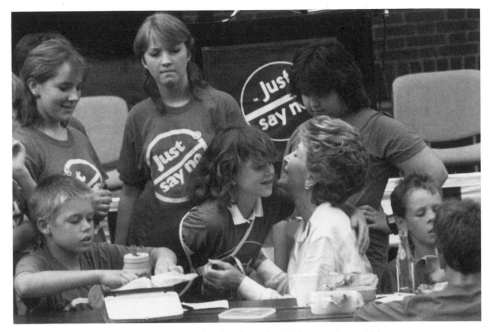

Former first lady Nancy Reagan promoting her "Just Say No" campaign, which encouraged children to choose not to start using drugs.

the addict "unlearn" the conditioned response of drug cravings. Psychologists call this the extinction of the conditioned response. A de-addicted person will no longer suffer from cravings for heroin and will be able to see old friends and acquaintances who were part of his or her "addicted life" without feeling the need to go back to it. De-addicted people will have enough outlets for stress and know how to relax and enjoy life in healthy ways so that drug use no longer has the same importance to them. Unfortunately, many addicts never reach this step. Most forms of recreation involve more effort and skill than drug use, and addicts may become discouraged at their difficulty.

The last step of successful recovery is the addict's personal realization that life is better without heroin, and a shift in values and perspectives that reflects this realization. Many recovered addicts experience this as a religious or spiritual awakening, with a sense of freedom from the pain and oppression of the addiction cycle and a reaffirmation of life and purpose. Heroin addiction attacks the very foundations of the human psyche, and complete recovery from its destructive power requires this reborn strength of spirit.

APPENDIX

FOR MORE INFORMATION

The following are good sources for information and help regarding heroin and drug abuse. There are also drug treatment programs and information hot lines listed in the telephone directories of almost every city, and local hospitals and medical centers often sponsor drug programs.

American Council for Drug Education
164 West 74th Street
New York, NY 10023
212-758-8060
1-800-448-DRUG

Hazelden Foundation/Pleasant Valley Road
P.O. Box 176
Center City, MN 55012
1-800-328-9000

Nar-Anon Family Groups
P.O. Box 2562
Palos Verdes Peninsula, CA 90274
310-547-5800

Narcotics Anonymous
P.O. Box 9999
Van Nuys, CA 91409
818-780-3951

National Clearinghouse for Alcohol and Drug Information
P.O. Box 2345
Rockville, MD 20847-2345
301-468-2600
1-800-729-6686

National Council on Alcoholism and Drug Dependence
12 West 21st Street, 7th Floor
New York, NY 10010
1-800-622-2255

National Families in Action
2296 Henderson Mill Road, Suite 300
Atlanta, GA 30345
404-934-6364

Center for Substance Abuse Treatment Information and Treatment Referral Hotline
11426-28 Rockville Pike, Suite 410
Rockville, MD 20852
1-800-662-HELP

APPENDIX

STATISTICS

TABLE 1: DRUG USER EXPENDITURES (in billions of dollars)

Drug	1988	1989	1990	1991	1992	1993	1994	1995
Cocaine	61.2	56.7	51.5	45.9	41.7	40.3	37.4	38.0
Heroin	17.7	16.8	14.3	11.9	10.2	9.8	9.3	9.6
Marijuana	9.1	10.9	11.0	10.7	11.5	8.8	8.2	7.0
Other	3.3	2.8	2.2	2.3	2.0	1.5	2.6	2.7
Totals	91.4	87.2	79.0	70.7	65.4	60.4	57.5	57.3

Note: Amounts are in constant 1996 dollars.
Source: Abt Associates, Inc., *What America's Users Spend on Illegal Drugs: 1988-1995* (November 1997).

TABLE 2: ESTIMATED NUMBER OF HARD-CORE AND OCCASIONAL USERS OF COCAINE AND HEROIN (Thousands), 1988-1995

Use	1988	1989	1990	1991	1992	1993	1994	1995
Cocaine								
Casual users (use less often than weekly)	6039	5313	4587	4478	3503	3332	2930	3082
Heavy users (use at least weekly)	4140	3889	3674	3501	3528	3598	3610	3620
Heroin								
Casual users (use less often than weekly)	167	152	136	172	207	199	206	322
Heavy users	876	881	784	730	692	787	799	810

Note: Data in this table are preliminary composite estimates from the National Household Survey on Drug Abuse (NHSDA) and the Drug Use Forecasting (DUF) program. The NHSDA was not administered in 1989. Estimates for 1989 are the average for 1988 and 1989.
Source: Abt Associates, Inc., *What America's Users Spend on Illicit Drugs: 1988-1995* (November 1997).

TABLE 3: PREVALENCE OF DRUG USE AMONG 6th-8th, 9th-12th, and 12th GRADE STUDENTS, 1994-95, 1995-96, and 1996-97

Annual Use	1994-95	1995-96	1996-97	Change*	Monthly Use	1994-95	1995-96	1996-97	Change*
Cigarettes					**Cigarettes**				
6th-8th	28.1	31.1	31.8	+0.7 s	6th-8th	15.7	17.2	17.3	+0.1
9th-12th	44.4	48.2	50.2	+2.0 s	9th-12th	31.3	33.4	34.7	+1.3 s
12th	46.8	50.0	52.4	+2.4 s	12th	34.6	36.2	38.3	+2.1 s
Beer					**Beer**				
6th-8th	30.8	33.1	33.2	+0.1	6th-8th	11.8	12.5	12.1	-0.4 s
9th-12th	57.4	59.1	59.6	+0.5 s	9th-12th	33.3	34.3	34.4	+0.1
12th	64.0	64.9	65.3	+0.4	12th	40.6	41.2	41.7	+0.5
Wine Coolers					**Wine Coolers**				
6th-8th	29.8	33.2	33.6	+0.4	6th-8th	9.8	10.8	10.8	+0.0
9th-12th	51.7	52.6	52.9	+0.3	9th-12th	23.1	22.3	22.3	+0.0
12th	56.5	54.5	55.4	+0.9	12th	25.6	22.9	23.7	+0.8
Liquor					**Liquor**				
6th-8th	21.3	22.9	23.7	+0.8 s	6th-8th	8.5	9.0	9.1	+0.1
9th-12th	51.5	53.4	54.9	+1.5 s	9th-12th	27.4	28.2	28.7	+0.5 s
12th	59.5	59.9	62.3	+2.4 s	12th	32.5	32.8	34.0	+1.2 s
Marijuana					**Marijuana**				
6th-8th	9.5	13.6	14.7	+1.1 s	6th-8th	5.7	8.1	8.6	+0.5 s
9th-12th	28.2	34.0	35.8	+1.8 s	9th-12th	18.5	22.3	22.7	+0.4
12th	33.2	37.9	39.4	+1.5 s	12th	20.9	24.3	24.4	+0.1
Cocaine					**Cocaine**				
6th-8th	1.9	2.7	3.0	+0.3 s	6th-8th	1.2	1.5	1.7	+0.2 s
9th-12th	4.5	5.6	5.9	+0.3 s	9th-12th	2.6	2.9	3.0	+0.1
12th	5.3	7.1	7.0	-0.1	12th	2.9	3.6	3.6	+0.0
Uppers					**Uppers**				
6th-8th	3.3	4.6	4.9	+0.3 s	6th-8th	2.0	2.4	2.6	+0.2 s
9th-12th	9.3	10.5	10.3	-0.2	9th-12th	5.1	5.2	5.3	+0.1
12th	10.6	11.6	10.7	-0.9 s	12th	5.6	5.8	5.6	-0.2
Downers					**Downers**				
6th-8th	2.4	3.5	4.0	+0.5 s	6th-8th	1.5	1.9	2.1	+0.2 s
9th-12th	5.5	7.1	7.2	+0.1	9th-12th	3.4	3.8	3.8	+0.0
12th	5.9	7.4	7.4	+0.0	12th	3.6	4.1	3.9	-0.2
Inhalants					**Inhalants**				
6th-8th	6.3	8.5	8.9	+0.4 s	6th-8th	2.9	3.5	3.7	+0.2
9th-12th	7.5	7.6	7.1	-0.5 s	9th-12th	3.5	3.4	3.1	-0.3 s
12th	6.6	6.6	5.8	-0.8 s	12th	3.0	3.1	2.7	-0.4 s
Hallucinogens					**Hallucinogens**				
6th-8th	2.4	3.3	3.6	+0.3 s	6th-8th	1.5	1.8	2.0	+0.2 s
9th-12th	7.7	9.5	9.5	+0.0	9th-12th	4.1	4.5	4.2	-0.3 s
12th	9.7	12.1	11.7	-0.4	12th	4.8	5.1	4.6	-0.5

* Note: Level of significance of difference between the 1995-96 and 1996-97 surveys: s=0.05, using chi-square with variables year and use/no use.

SAMPLE SIZES:	Grade	1994-95	1995-96	1996-97
	6th-8th	92,453	58,596	68,071
	9th-12th	105,788	70,964	73,006
	12th	20,698	14,261	15,532

Source: PRIDE USA Survey 1994–95, 1995–96, and 1996–97.

TABLE 4: PERCENTAGE REPORTING HEROIN USE IN THEIR LIFETIME, BY AGE GROUP AND DEMOGRAPHIC CHARACTERISTICS: 1995

Demographic Characteristic	Age Group (Years) 12-17	18-25	26-34	35+	Total
Total	0.7	0.7	1.5	1.2	1.2
Gender					
Male	0.7	0.7	1.9	2.2	1.8
Female	0.6	0.8	1.0	0.4	0.6
Race/Ethnicity[1]					
White	0.8	1.0	1.6	1.1	1.1
Black	*	0.3	0.8	3.3	1.9
Hispanic	0.4	0.2	1.3	0.7	0.7
Population Density					
Large Metro	1.0	0.6	1.3	1.2	1.1
Small Metro	0.6	1.2	1.5	1.3	1.2
Nonmetro	0.3	0.4	1.7	1.3	1.1
Region					
Northeast	0.3	1.0	1.3	1.6	1.4
North Central	1.4	0.8	0.7	1.1	1.0
South	0.4	0.9	1.4	1.5	1.3
West	0.5	0.4	2.4	0.7	1.0
Adult Education[2]					
Less than high school	N/A	1.2	2.6	0.7	1.1
High school graduate	N/A	1.1	1.0	1.2	1.2
Some college	N/A	0.3	2.2	1.7	1.5
College graduate	N/A	*	0.8	1.3	1.1
Current Employment[3]					
Full-time	N/A	0.7	1.1	1.5	1.3
Part-time	N/A	0.8	2.1	1.2	1.2
Unemployed	N/A	2.1	3.1	*	4.0
Other[4]	N/A	0.3	1.9	0.6	0.7

*Low precision; no estimate reported

N/A: Not applicable

Note: Due to improved procedures implemented in 1994, these estimates are not comparable to those presented in NHSDA Main Findings prior to 1994.

[1] The category "other" for Race/Ethnicity is not included.

[2] Data on adult education are not applicable for youth age 12-17. Total refers to adults age 18 and older (unweighted N=13, 152).

[3] Data on current employment are not applicable for youth age 12-17. Total refers to adults age 18 and older (unweighted N=13, 152).

[4] Retired, disabled, homemaker, student, or "other."

Source: Office of Applied Studies, SAMHSA, National Household Survey on Drug Abuse, 1995.

APPENDIX

GLOSSARY

Delirium: a disturbance of consciousness and thought processes, characterized by an inability to focus, sustain, or shift attention; susceptibility to distraction by irrelevant stimuli; and reduced awareness of one's surroundings.

Detoxification: the process of removing drugs and other chemicals from the body. Also, any treatment program designed to help a person undergo that process.

Endorphins: protein compounds released by the pituitary gland that act as natural painkillers and cause a feeling of euphoria. Endorphins are released when the body is in pain, or after prolonged exercise. They attach to the same receptors in the brain as chemicals like morphine and heroin.

Heroin: the trade name given to diacetylmorphine, one of the strongest of the opiate drugs. Heroin is known by many street names, including "H," "horse," "smack," and "junk."

Intoxication: the changes in a person's physical or mental state brought on by the presence of drugs in the body. Opioid intoxication can include such symptoms as mood changes, apathy, impaired judgment, drowsiness, slurred speech, impairment of attention or memory, and markedly speeded or slowed muscular activity.

Methadone: a synthetic opioid developed in Germany during World War II as a substitute for morphine. Methadone produces less intense but longer-lasting effects than heroin or morphine.

Methadone maintenance: a treatment for long-term addicts whose body chemistry requires the presence of opioids, in which prescribed doses of methadone are given once per day.

Morphine: an opiate developed at the beginning of the 19th century, used first for its painkilling properties and later as a recreational drug before its addictive properties were understood.

Naloxene/naltrexone: opiate antagonists used in a new, controversial rapid detoxification system to help addicts complete the detoxification and withdrawal process within hours instead of weeks.

Opiate/opioid: generic terms for all drugs derived from the opium poppy, or synthesized to have similar effect. Opiates are specifically those derived from the plant, while opioids include both natural and synthetic forms of the drug.

Opioid antagonist: a drug, such as naloxene or naltrexone, that stimulates the body to purge opioids from its system. These drugs frequently cause violent withdrawal symptoms.

Opioid receptors: the parts of the brain that process endorphins and also process opioid drugs like heroin and morphine.

Physical dependence: the adaptation of body chemistry to require regular doses of a drug for normal functioning. Opioids can cause severe physical dependence.

Psychological dependence: the development of strong cravings to use a drug, even if there is no physical urge to do so. Opioids cause severe psychological dependence.

Psychotic disorder: a mental condition in which a person suffers from delusions and/or hallucinations. Frequently, when accompanying use of heroin or other opioids, this disorder includes the delusion of being persecuted.

Substance-induced disorder: a mental problem, such as a mood disorder, delirium, or psychotic disorder, that is caused by the use of drugs.

Substance-use disorder: the unhealthy use of a drug or the effects of that use. Opioid dependence and opioid abuse are substance-use disorders.

Tolerance: the addict's need for increasing amounts of a drug to achieve the same level of intoxication. Long-term addicts may develop such high tolerance that they can take amounts that would kill a non-user.

Withdrawal: the physical and mental symptoms that occur when a person who is physically dependent on a drug stops taking the drug. Withdrawal symptoms include physical distress similar to a bad case of the flu, including muscle aches and cramps, fever, vomiting, and weakness, as well as mental symptoms such as depression and hallucinations.

APPENDIX

BIBLIOGRAPHY

American Psychiatric Association. *Diagnostic and Statistical Manual of Mental Disorders*, 4th ed. Washington, D.C.: American Psychiatric Press, 1994.

Courtwright, David. *Dark Paradise: Opiate Addiction in America before 1940.* Cambridge: Harvard University Press, 1982.

Cox, Christopher. *Chasing the Dragon: Into the Heartland of the Golden Triangle.* New York: Henry Holt, 1997.

Hanson, William. *Life with Heroin: Voices from the Inner City.* Lexington, Mass.: Lexington Books, 1985.

Hutchings, Donald. *Methadone: Treatment for Addiction.* New York: Chelsea House Publishers, 1992.

Kaplan, John. *The Hardest Drug: Heroin and Public Policy.* Chicago: University of Chicago Press, 1985.

Lockley, Paul. *Counselling Heroin and Other Drug Users.* New York: New York University Press, 1995.

McCoy, Alfred W. *The Politics of Heroin: CIA Complicity in the Global Drug Trade.* New York: Lawrence Hill & Co., 1991

Trebach, Arnold. *The Heroin Solution.* New Haven: Yale University Press, 1982.

Zackon, Fred. *Heroin: The Street Narcotic.* New York: Chelsea House Publishers, 1992.

APPENDIX

INDEX

APPENDIX

PICTURE CREDITS

Senior Consulting Editor Carol C. Nadelson, M.D., is president and chief executive officer of the American Psychiatric Press, Inc., staff physician at Cambridge Hospital, and Clinical Professor of Psychiatry at Harvard Medical School. In addition to her work with the American Psychiatric Association, which she served as vice president in 1981–83 and president in 1985–86, Dr. Nadelson has been actively involved in other major psychiatric organizations, including the Group for the Advancement of Psychiatry, the American College of Psychiatrists, the Association for Academic Psychiatry, the American Association of Directors of Psychiatric Residency Training Programs, the American Psychosomatic Society, and the American College of Mental Health Administrators. In addition, she has been a consultant to the Psychiatric Education Branch of the National Institute of Mental Health and has served on the editorial boards of several journals. Doctor Nadelson has received many awards, including the Gold Medal Award for significant and ongoing contributions in the field of psychiatry, the Elizabeth Blackwell Award for contributions to the causes of women in medicine, and the Distinguished Service Award from the American College of Psychiatrists for outstanding achievements and leadership in the field of psychiatry.

Consulting Editor Claire E. Reinburg, M.A., is editorial director of the American Psychiatric Press, Inc., which publishes about 60 new books and six journals a year. She is a graduate of Georgetown University in Washington, D.C., where she earned bachelor of arts and master of arts degrees in English. She is a member of the Council of Biology Editors, the Women's National Book Association, the Society for Scholarly Publishing, and Washington Book Publishers.

Ann Holmes has written and edited professionally for over 15 years. Her special areas of interest are both cultural and medical topics. Her books include *The Psychological Effects of Cocaine and Crack Addiction* in Chelsea House Publishers' ENCYCLOPEDIA OF PSYCHOLOGICAL DISORDERS. Ann and her family live in southwestern Pennsylvania, where she edits *The Loyalhanna Review*, the literary journal of the Ligonier Valley Writers.